SEX IN A TENT

SEX IN A TENT

A Wild Couple's Guide to Getting Naughty in Nature

By Michelle Waitzman

 WILDERNESS PRESS · BERKELEY, CA

Sex in a Tent:
A Wild Couple's Guide to Getting Naughty in Nature

1st EDITION November 2007
  2nd printing May 2008

Copyright © 2007 by Michelle Waitzman

Illustrations: Ann Miya
Book design: Jeremy Stout
Book editor: Eva Dienel

Library of Congress Card Number: 2007016839
ISBN: 978-0-89997-432-3
UPC: 7-19609-97432-1

Manufactured in China

Published by: **Wilderness Press**
  1200 5th Street
  Berkeley, CA 94710
  (800) 443-7227; FAX (510) 558-1696
  info@wildernesspress.com
  www.wildernesspress.com

Visit our website for a complete listing of our books
and for ordering information.

Library of Congress Cataloging-in-Publication Data

Waitzman, Michelle.
  Sex in a tent : a wild couple's guide to getting naughty in nature /
  Michelle Waitzman. — 1st ed.
    p. cm.
  Includes bibliographical references and index.
  ISBN 978-0-89997-432-3
  1. Sex—Miscellanea. 2. Camping—Miscellanea. 3. Outdoor recre-
  ation—Miscellanea. I. Title.
  HQ23.W17 2007
  306.709173'4—dc22   2007016839

ACKNOWLEDGMENTS

For Gerhard

There are many people without whom this book would simply not have been written. I'd like to take this opportunity to thank them for making it possible. First, Matt Wagner of Fresh Books Literary Agency, who was willing to take a chance on a first-timer, which is rare these days. Roslyn Bullas and Eva Dienel at Wilderness Press, who showed so much enthusiasm for this project that it made me want to work harder to live up to their expectations. My supportive friends, Tobey, Gill, Rosie, Francine, and Reg, who, despite our physical distance, are always there for me. My parents, Emile and Suzy, who always manage to be proud of me, no matter how strange my accomplishments. Gerhard, who is always there with a hug and a positive outlook—you're both the angel over my right shoulder and the devil over my left! Thanks also to all of the people who were willing to share their camping experiences and stories with me, and are celebrated throughout the book. This book is about you, so keep on enjoying the great outdoors together!

CONTENTS

Introduction:

How Camping Can

IMPROVE
YOUR
SEX LIFE

I know what you're thinking: How could a book on camping possibly improve your sex life? Admittedly, it sounds unlikely. For most, camping is about challenging ourselves against nature, with only a thin layer of Gore-Tex to protect us from the elements. Traditionally, people went into the woods to tough it out, not to get it on. Most likely, your idea of a romantic weekend away involves crisp linens and room service—and there's nothing wrong with that. But once in a while, even the bottle of sparkling chilling in a stand next to the rose-petal-covered bed in your five-star hotel gets a little mundane. Maybe you and your lover are ready for something different. Something wilder. Something outside the walls of your bedroom. Something just plain *outside.*

The exhilaration of the wilderness can really fan our flames when it comes to love. In reality, the pursuits of the great outdoors and great sex are not all that different. Think about what people look for in great sex: spontaneity, adventure, mystery, excitement, uncertainty. If you asked Sir Edmund Hillary why he "mounted" Everest, he just might give you the same list.

If your sex life is lacking excitement, the problem might be the scenery, not the performers. Camping together will definitely change the scenery. After all, it's something we do to put some adventure back into our lives—and if you believe the dozens of best-selling books, talk shows, and advice columns on improving your sex life, adventure is the one thing we could all use a bit more of between the sheets.

Consider Heather, an Arizona camper who is so enthusiastic about her outdoor escapades that she maintains a website entitled "Naked in the Woods." Heather and her husband, John, make it a point to "play naked" whenever possible on their outdoor adventures. In their nine years of camping together, they have had sex on the top of a mountain, on hiking trails, in the water, and, of course, on a beach. According to Heather, the whole idea of

being someplace where they could get caught is enough to keep them seeking out more romantic adventures on our public lands. And indeed, she says, "We've been caught many, many times! That just makes it more exciting!"

Not everyone is so comfortable with public exposure, but these two have found the perfect way to rejuvenate their sex life by taking it away from their regular routine. According to Esther Perel, a therapist who counsels couples in the urban wilds of New York, the domestic comforts of home can be a real turnoff. In her book, *Mating in Captivity: Reconciling the Erotic + the Domestic* (HarperCollins 2006), Perel looks at the things that can get in the way of erotic desire for long-term couples. She thinks it's a great idea to trade mating in captivity for mating in the wild now and then. With no bedroom, no TV, no phone, and no schedule, you'll be free to let your imagination take over.

"We tend to associate home with the place where you feel serious and responsible; it's not a place we associate with playfulness," Perel says. "You can make home predictable, but you can't make nature predictable. It can bring out playfulness. When you go into nature, you go to play."

That sense of adventure and play is what gives sex its spark. And the more challenges you face in the wild together, the hotter the results. Climb a mountain with your lover , and you may find your libido rising right along with the elevation. "At home, there's nothing to defy, to resist, to conquer," says Perel. "Home is comfortable, it's easy. Nature adds an edge."

Priya, a nature-lover from South Africa, couldn't agree more with Perel's theories. "Worry is a great passion killer, and as nature relaxes you, chances are just much more favorable for romance," she says. "In addition to that, usually you have far fewer distractions and responsibilities when you're out camping; therefore you have more time to spend together, which is usually very limited in any work day." Priya even finds the exertions

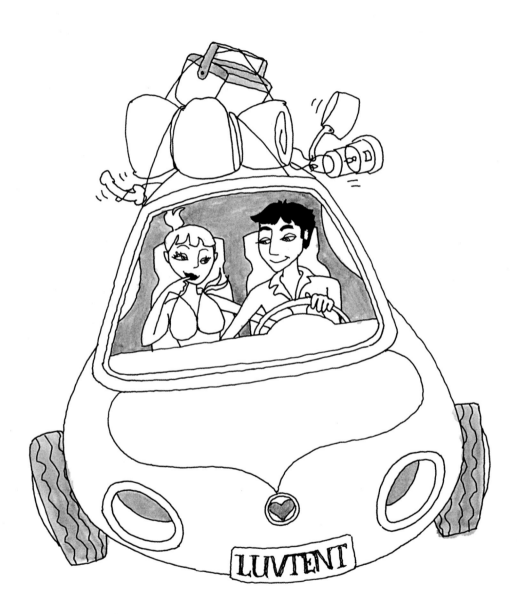

of camping sexy. "The working up a sweat and getting physical relates to exactly what you'd be doing in the bedroom, not so?"

Kathleen Meyer, a longtime outdoorswoman and author (she wrote the popular tome *How to Shit in the Woods*, about the *other* call of nature), has all but abandoned her traditional bedroom. She and her partner, Patrick McCarron, love the outdoors so much that even at home they prefer to sleep outside on their uncovered deck. "The air feels so good compared to the indoor air," Meyer says. "And having the sky open to you is tremendous. We watch the sky at night, and we know a lot of the constellations—they're like friends up there. It kind of puts you in closer touch with the universe and makes you feel more a part of it."

Not many of us can bring our camping practices home like they do, but imagine how wonderful it would be to snuggle in your double sleeping bag every night, enjoying fresh air and a starry sky together. When Meyer and McCarron do leave their Montana home and venture deep into the wilderness, it gives them an even greater thrill. "There's nobody but us and the wolves and the moose up there," Meyer says. "And just to feel the world as your own, to be that isolated, I find that thrilling."

While Meyer and McCarron seem to have it all worked out, I have to admit that my own first experiences mixing camping with romance didn't quite live up to my wildest fantasies. Mostly they involved a lot of muffling noises with body parts, Therm-a-Rest rug burn, and some rather inconvenient cramping. But I just knew that if I could get beyond the "technical difficulties," there would be plenty of excitement and hot adventures waiting for me.

One morning, after a particularly unsatisfying night in the woods, I declared that there ought to be a book about how to have sex in a tent. It wasn't until later that it occurred to me to write the book myself. Now, after a lot of fulfilling "research," I am making it my mission to bring passion and romance to campers everywhere. I'm here to tell you that camping doesn't just bring you closer to nature, it brings you closer to each other. It's time to check out a whole new world of nature at its naughtiest!

Great Sex and the Great Outdoors

Consider your usual love life at home. If you're like most of us, it gets squeezed in between working too much, making dinner, shopping, taking care of the kids, mowing the lawn, and a million other boring tasks. If you're lucky, you've set aside a date night when you regularly have sex in the bedroom after dinner and a movie. The lights are out, and you're on auto-pilot. It's hard to be inspired when everything around you is so familiar and predictable.

Now consider your relationship outside of that bedroom box. Imagine spending a whole day walking hand in hand through the forest, flirting like you did when you first met. Picture your protective instincts kicking in when you think you might be lost. Connect with your most primitive passions and imagine lying in a pile of fallen leaves, naked with your soul mate (or perhaps your first date). It's not your usual Saturday night in—and it's bound to take you places you don't normally go.

Venturing into the wilderness with your partner creates a different dynamic in your relationship. You'll have to throw away the typical gender roles. Women will have to pull their weight when it comes to carrying gear, and men will have to help out with dinner. And if you want to take a break from your regular roles during sex, well, that's not a bad idea, either. Maybe it's the lady's turn to talk dirty. Perhaps your bandana would make a handy blindfold. Here's your chance to push your boundaries and try something new.

Couples therapist Perel sees camping as a time when partners can really shake up the way they relate. "There's something that goes beyond gender, into competencies and sensibilities," she explains. "If one partner is more competent at home, but in nature, the other is more competent and has the power, the roles have shifted because he is at ease in that environment. So people who are shy at home might be more daring when they're camping."

For Kiwi camping enthusiast Justine, the "rough and ready" version of her man is a total turn-on. "There's nothing sexier than seeing your partner happy in the bush with a streak of mud on his face," she says.

It's no surprise that we get the hots for our partners when we see this survivalist streak in them. It's a matter of looking at someone you know all too well in a new light. Maybe you're accustomed to seeing your guy lazing on the couch watching the game; when you watch him rigging a makeshift shelter, it's a bit like discovering an endangered species. It's intriguing and thrilling at the same time—is this really *my* man? "Very often, people are most attracted when their partner's 'otherness' is accentuated—when they are competent doing things you can't do," Perel says. "There is a mystery—you see them from a distance. He's doing something that is his that has nothing to do with me." Whether it's catching fish for dinner or climbing a rock face, it feels great to remember why you admire the one you love.

My friend Maria recently got into a relationship with an outdoorsman. At first she was nervous about joining his adventures, but once she gave it a try, she found his wild side very attractive. "He is gorgeous at any time, but there is something about the wind in his hair, the color the mountain air puts in his cheeks, the effort of the exercise that makes him completely irresistible," she says. Seeing him so confident in the wilderness is part of his appeal. "He's spent a lot of time outdoors, doing some, what I would call 'extreme' sports (though I'm sure he would deny that they were extreme), and so he feels comfortable and happy during our trips," Maria adds.

For me, sometimes it's my own outdoorsy side that provides the spark. I feel so confident and inspired when I get to the end of a tough trail or reach the top of a mountain, that my self-esteem soars. Feeling so great about myself translates into feeling strong and sexy. I'm rarely the sexual aggressor at home, but inside the tent, I'm ready to say I've earned it! It's not just the boys who look good with a bit of dirt under their fingernails.

Camping as a Couple

When I surveyed couples for this book, I was surprised by how many of them simply didn't have a sex life when they went camping. There are people who think of camping as something to do with their buddies, so when they camp, they tend to treat their partner the same way— like a buddy.

Your buddies may think it's hilarious when you pee over the side of the canoe, but your wife is less likely to be amused. I've been on group trips where the guys belched and farted around the campfire like it was half the fun of being there. The girls just rolled their eyes. The men needed to stop and think about how they behave on camping trips, and compare it to how they usually act around their partners. I'm willing to bet that none of those women was in a big hurry to have hot sex with her guy that night.

Suffice to say, bringing together your love life and your love of the outdoors may be a bit of an adjustment. Lifelong campers usually start out considering it an asexual hobby—more about toughing it out than indulging their fantasies. But spending time outside is a sensual experience. People go into the woods to awaken their senses— to feel the wind on their faces, to breathe the clean, fresh air, and to let the sun warm their skin. Jessica, a camper from Michigan, told me that she thinks it's perfectly natural for those highly sensual feelings to add romance to her camping trips.

"All of your senses are alive in nature," she says. "Being out in the woods is a natural buzz anyway, but there's

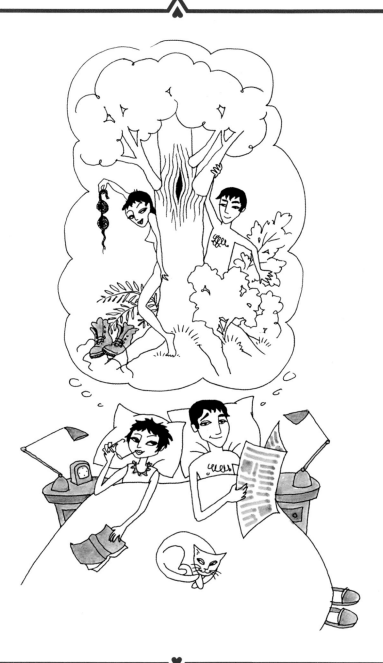

something about being 'wild and free' with your partner. There is nothing more romantic than cuddling with my husband under a sky full of stars, or waking up in the perfect quiet of dawn."

Camping can be about indulging your senses, but it can also be a romantically indulgent experience. No longer is it all about denying yourself luxuries and suffering against the elements with the barest of essentials. Camping has discovered decadence! Even the outdoor gear and clothing companies sense the romance in the air. You don't have to shop at Victoria's Secret for thong underwear; you can buy it from Patagonia. And what better place to show it off than in MSR's two-person tent, the Hubba Hubba? They've also got a model called the Fling—proving once and for all that even mountaineers have time for a quickie. When you're ready to commit to your outdoor love life, you can pick up REI's wedding cake topper featuring a couple in mountain-climbing gear. (That outdoor retailer has even introduced a wedding registry service, where you can order things like backcountry margarita glasses and even a Lexan blender to make cocktails.) Couples everywhere are making it clear that camping is a big part of their relationships.

"Our industry has been asleep when it comes to sexiness," admits Beaver Theodosakis, founder and president of Prana, the outdoor clothing company that had the groundbreaking idea of outfitting sexy climber bodies with equally sexy clothing. "I think that's hurt the industry. The way the advertising used to be a picture of a guy out on a mountain by himself with ice in his beard. In our catalogs and ads, we try to show a more playful attitude, with guys and girls interacting and natural sexiness." Yes, even mountain men have love lives these days.

Shifting your point of view to consider camping as a couple opens up a whole new world of possibilities. Couples who go camping together often find it improves their level of trust, their closeness, their ability to solve problems together, and their sex lives. One camper from New Zealand, Hillary, found that she could discuss things with her husband during camping trips that they would never talk about at home. Somehow, being outside makes him more open to conversation. For a lot of men, it comes down to feeling "in their element" out in the woods. For many women, leaving behind the worries of home and work makes the outdoors a great place to reconnect as well. It's an environment where a couple can really come together. Getting back to basics while camping can bring you back to the basics of your relationship, too.

Heather, the camper from Arizona, finds that her husband can relax more in the wild. "When we're camping together, what I like most about John is that he's much more carefree and laidback," she says. "He's not 'at work' anymore." Camping is their time to be close, Heather says. "We each have our separate things that we do: John skydives, and I do things like scrapbooking and spending time with my friends. But together, we have this passion for the outdoors that we share."

This is true for a lot of couples. At home, two people can lead very separate lives, even under the same roof. But camping can give them the time and inspiration to really enjoy each other's company. "I'm a writer, he's into computers," says Justine "We hate each other's taste in music, clothes, houses, possessions. But it doesn't matter if we can come together the way we do when we're camping. I'm just living each moment, with the man I love, in the most beautiful mountains in the world. That's very fresh and simple somehow. There's just a calm that you're in the right place, sharing it with the right person."

Once you have started to camp as a couple, it's something you can do together for the rest of your lives. It's inexpensive, the gear lasts for years, and as long as you have transportation, you can enjoy a camping trip at any time. Jessica told me she recently met a couple who are traveling around the US, doing a lot of camping now that their kids have all grown up and moved out. "They are enjoying each other and the country so much," she says wistfully. "I can't wait till we can do the same…in a couple of decades."

I often come across couples well into their 70s enjoying a hike through the woods or a paddle on their favorite lake. The best thing about it is seeing that romantic sparkle in their eyes. Getting outdoors together keeps them young and passionate well into their golden years. The playwright George Bernard Shaw once said, "We don't stop playing because we grow old. We grow old because we stop playing." So keep playing outside with your partner, and you'll stay young forever!

About this Book

As you have probably already guessed, this is not your average camping book. You won't find anything here about navigating with a map and compass, or building an emergency shelter out of branches—unless you're doing it for sexual role-playing purposes (there's nothing like a little game of *Survivor*), in which case, may I suggest tying the supports together with a strong rope so you don't have a mid-coitus collapse. This book is about making your outdoor experiences more romantic and sexier than you've ever imagined.

Throughout this book, you'll read stories from couples who will give you a peek at their secrets to wilderness romance. I've maintained their anonymity and changed some details and names for obvious reasons—you never know whose mother might be reading—except where they've specifically wanted their name in lights. (And with some of their stories, who wouldn't be proud!)

Chapter by chapter, we'll look at how to introduce an absolute beginner to camping, how to plan your camping trips so that you both enjoy them, how to keep yourselves clean and attractive in the wilderness, how to make gourmet meals for two without a kitchen, how to approach different kinds of camping for maximum romance, where to go for the ultimate wilderness getaways, and, of course, how to have sex in a tent and just about anywhere else outdoors.

In order to keep things simple, this book generally refers to couples as one man and one woman. This by no means suggests that same-sex couples can't use this book as a guide for planning their own romantic outdoor adventures. All couples will find that their relationship changes when they leave the comforts of home behind, regardless of gender. For the most part, there will be very little difference in terms of the challenges and rewards you will face. In places where same-sex couples may encounter their own unique situations, I'll address them separately.

Ideally, both members of a couple should read this book. If you'll excuse the pun, it will keep you on the same page when it comes to planning your camping adventures. If only one of you reads it, you can share with your partner the ideas you'd like to try. Bring them up over dinner, or on a lazy weekend. Get your partner excited about the idea of camping together, be sure to mention all of the amazing sex you'll be having, then pick a time to get out there and give it a shot.

I sincerely believe that even the most urban of us can get into camping just by being open to the experience. But having a supportive and enthusiastic partner makes it so much easier and more enjoyable. So I encourage you to try it out—it's good for you, it's good for your relationship, and as you'll see in this book, it's good for your sex life, too!

Chapter 1:

Convincing Your Reluctant Partner that
CAMPING IS FUN

I wasn't born into camping. We never went as a family because my father firmly believed that if you own a perfectly good bed, you should use it. So, I have to admit that before I started camping, I had some pretty crazy ideas of what it might be like. I thought that you had to find your way around with a map and a compass in the wild, because I didn't know about trail markers. I thought you had to be able to make a fire in the rain to cook your food, because I'd never seen a camping stove. I thought there would be bugs crawling around inside the tent all night—and I had a huge bug phobia. Suffice to say, the idea that camping might be romantic never entered my mind.

When you've been doing the camping thing for a while, it's easy to forget that not everybody is familiar with the way things work in the woods. And when you're worried about staying alive, you tend to put passion on the backburner. If you're introducing a newcomer to camping, don't make any assumptions about what that person knows.

For true city-slickers, it's like being beamed up to another planet—and it can be downright intimidating. When Hillary met her future husband, she wasn't a camper. He, however, had been camping with his family since he was little. "The only question they ever had to settle was whether to head for the mountains or the beach," says Hillary. "But it wasn't a holiday unless they packed up the tent and crammed the whole family into the car to set up at a campground somewhere."

Hillary knew it would mean a lot to him if she tried his favorite pastime, but she was willing to do so on one condition: He had to do all the work. "I just trusted him to take care of everything, and, in fact, he still does," says Hillary, who is now a camping convert. "Camping is a real vacation for me because he does absolutely everything—cooking, cleaning, and organizing."

While at first camping was a big adjustment, Hillary soon figured out the trick for her was to avoid comparing it to the way things are at home. A few bugs weren't the end of the world, even if she found one in her tea.

Her willingness to give camping a shot made all the difference in their relationship. "The fact that I had a good time on our first trip may have been the key to our entire relationship from that day forward," she says. "It's hard to say. But we go on a trip every three months and we've been doing it for years."

Hillary and her husband are a good example of how to get a novice to go camping. If you are introducing your partner to camping, be sure to take your partner's concerns seriously, and deal with them before you go on your first camping trip. If you're the beginner, make sure you speak up about the things that are worrying you. You can't expect your partner to predict everything that might make you nervous. Don't be afraid that your partner will think you're being stupid or wimpy—you aren't supposed to know everything the first time out. Remember: If both of you are comfortable with what's going on, camping together will be fun for each of you, and you might even be able to indulge in some of the romantic stuff.

Start with the Good Stuff

Sure, there are fears and difficulties to deal with, but let's begin by looking at all of the great things about camping together. It's going to be a whole lot easier to talk your partner into trying it out if you can provide some tempting reasons. (And if you're the non-camper, listen up!)

Try this for starters: "Honey, if we go camping, you can have a whole weekend without hearing the phone ring, or de-spamming your email, or checking off chores on your to-do list. It will just be you and me, with no interruptions. We can do whatever we want, whenever we want. Doesn't that sound nice?"

What couple couldn't use a little more alone time these days? Leaving your usual life behind is a great way to refresh things between you and deepen your relationship. If that doesn't work, crank it up a notch: "Baby, going out into the woods brings out the wild beast in me! I just want to get you out there alone so we can run naked through the grass and keep the animals awake all night while we howl at the moon." Who could turn down an invitation like that?

If your partner is a romantic, don't forget to mention the opportunities for cuddling by the campfire, eating dinner by moonlight, and skinny dipping under the stars. If it sounds like fun, not work, you'll have a much easier time making it happen.

Camping together can make your relationship stronger by giving you a deeper trust in one another. You will be

Top 10 Reasons to Camp Together

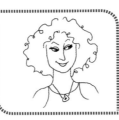

Is your partner still not convinced? Try my top 10 list. These reasons always work for me!

1. See wildlife without paying zoo admission.
2. Walk all day breathing pollution-free air.
3. See how bright the stars really are.
4. Have conversations that last longer than commercial breaks.
5. Wake up to the sun, not the alarm clock.
6. Toast marshmallows over a campfire.
7. Actually enjoy getting exercise.
8. Hold hands all day.
9. Enjoy dining al fresco.
10. Go skinny dipping!

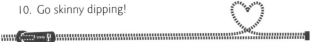

physically challenged, have to adapt to changing conditions, and find ways to get by with no help from the outside world. It's amazing when you realize that the only person you need to survive is your partner. Learning to solve your problems together in the wild makes problems at home seem much more manageable. Knowing you can work through any situation together is going to make you a more confident, more dedicated "team."

Kathleen Meyer, a prominent outdoor writer from Montana who also used to guide rafting trips, has experienced the joy of bringing new campers into the wild, and watching their self-esteem grow as they master new skills. "It's that self-esteem that you build when you're doing things that you haven't done before and facing situations that are new to you," she says. "You bring that confidence back to the city with you. In a relationship, it builds that mutual confidence in your togetherness, that you have survived something, so that it becomes a bonding."

Even if you do encounter difficulties while camping— and chances are, you will at some point—dealing with those challenges might be the best way to bring you and your lover closer. It's no coincidence that war buddies have some of the strongest friendships. It's the challenges we overcome together that build connections. When you begin to admire someone for what you've seen them do, it's easy for that admiration to become something more. Friendship? Lust? Love? When we're camping, we intentionally put ourselves into challenging situations, so the odds of admiring each other at the end of the day are pretty good. And then we get to crawl into the tent and express our admiration in all kinds of fun ways.

Going camping as a couple can also give you a shared feeling of accomplishment. Nothing is better than standing at the summit of a mountain (even a small one) with someone you love, knowing that the two of you made it up there the hard way. I defy you not to top it off with a big, heartfelt kiss! It's one of the most popular places for hikers to propose marriage. How could you possibly say no with all of those endorphins running through your body?

One of the things that is so addictive about camping is the wonderful scenery you get to see along the way. Untouched wilderness, spectacular views, and sparkling lakes are just a few of the joys of getting away from civilization. Seeing these things with someone you love makes them even more special, because they become part of your shared experience as a couple. You can look at a picture and be transported back to a moment in time without saying a word. You can mention a particularly hot night of sex you had on a trip, and know that the place will forever mean something different to you than to anyone else who goes there.

Ross Morton, who works with the outdoor education program Outward Bound, says it's a matter of recognizing those magical moments so you can take them in together. "Even though you may be focused on the end (goal), or what you're doing, moments of beauty can stop people in their tracks," he says. When two people stop to share one of those moments of beauty, sparks will fly.

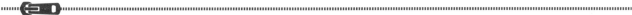

High-Altitude
Pick-Up Artist

66 Several years ago, a guy friend—let's call him Don Juan—invited me to climb Mt. Whitney with him. I was fairly new to California, and as an outdoorsy girl, I looked forward to climbing the state's highest peak. I really had no romantic interest in Don whatsoever, so it caught me off-guard when, about halfway up to our base camp at Upper Boy Scout Lake, he broached the subject of whether we might make a good couple. I didn't want to hurt his feelings, or ruin our shot at the summit, so I gave him the I-really-don't-want-to-ruin-our-friendship line.

I figured Don had gotten the hint because when we were filtering water at camp that afternoon, he took note of my pink toenail polish and told me he was more attracted to women who had the "natural" look, anyway. (I briefly considered using one of my painted-toenail feet to kick him in the butt, but then I figured it was in my best interest that he was no longer attracted to me.)

Later that night, however, Don must have forgotten his aversion to my nail polish. Just minutes after I snuggled into my sleeping bag in our shared tent, I felt his hand gently stroke the length of my body. I ignored him and scooted closer to my side of the tent. Then he did it again. Once more, I ignored him. But he needed an answer. "Eh-hem," Don said, matter-of-factly. "How would you feel about a little non-committal cuddling?"

I toyed with the idea of asking him exactly what that meant: Did his no-nail polish rule have a high-altitude sex clause? Instead, I simply told him, "No thanks," and curled up to sleep.

The next morning, we climbed Whitney without a hitch, and I felt relieved until I realized that I had plans to go on a climbing trip with him and a group of mutual friends the very next weekend. As a safeguard, I brought my two dogs. When he asked whether he could share my tent, I motioned to the dogs and said, "Sorry, it's full." I have to admit, I felt a bit sorry for him when he realized my dogs were the only ones who would get any "heavy petting" that night. **99**

—*ED*

Deal with the Scary Stuff

It may be a little hard to concentrate on these moments of beauty if one of you is actually afraid you'll be attacked by a bear at any minute. Putting your partner at ease before the first trip will leave you free to really enjoy yourselves. Once you know how to overcome possible problems, they won't seem like such a big deal anymore.

It's important to go into the wilderness feeling confident and prepared, particularly the first time. So let's look at some common fears for first-time or inexperienced campers, and how you can make them less of a concern.

Remember, just because something doesn't worry you doesn't mean that it's unreasonable for your partner to be scared. I used to be so freaked out by bugs that if I saw a centipede crawl across the floor, I'd go running out of the room. My boyfriend at the time thought I was nuts. "What do think that centipede is going to do to you?" I had no rational answer, but the fact is, my heart would start to pound, and when I saw just one bug, it was like I could feel a million of them crawling all over me. That was just an irrational fear of something that couldn't really hurt me, but there are some very, very rational fears associated with going camping.

Kathleen Meyer's attempts at introducing city boys to river rafting caused her a lot of grief in her love life. Somehow, she just couldn't see that they were frightened by the rapids. "I really don't know what happened," she says. "I think I probably blew a lot of them away. I don't know if it was the wilderness or the rapids or just my choices (of men)."

Assuming that your partner is comfortable right away will often lead to problems. When it's the woman who is the experienced one, it's easy to forget that a beginner is a beginner—even if he's a man. "For me, it would be a role reversal to pamper a man in a way that might make him feel more comfortable out there, the way men typically do for women," Meyer says. "I'd expect the man to be ready and up for the wilderness, more so than I am,

I guess." She learned the hard way that anyone can be scared doing a new activity, even if he seems tough in his everyday life.

You or your partner may have fears or concerns about camping that I don't cover in this section. Make sure you talk about them together, and find ways of dealing with them before you make your first trip. Respecting your partner's opinions is important if you want to have a trusting relationship. If you deal with any potential problems ahead of time, you can spend your trip focused on the fun stuff.

Wild Animals

On my very first camping trip, our group returned from a swim down at the beach to find a black bear at our campsite sniffing around the tents. Someone must have left food around. I knew nothing about bears, so when one of the leaders starting yelling at the bear and clapping her hands, I thought she was crazy. He's going to come and attack us if you yell like that!

If you're taking a beginner somewhere with bears, wolves, coyotes, or other wild beasts, make sure you give them some background knowledge first. If you're a new camper with concerns, ask your partner or talk with the local ranger about whether any native wildlife pose a danger. Now I know you're supposed to make noise so you don't surprise the bear, because that's when they charge. But that would have been a good thing to know before I saw one. Let your partner know how to handle wild animal encounters, and what precautions you should both be taking. If the beginner knows that tying up the food and garbage between trees will keep the bears away from the tent, he or she will probably get a much better night's sleep.

Snakes are classic phobia-inspiring creatures. Even experienced campers can be caught off guard when they run across a snake. I was doing a guided desert hike in Arizona's Vermilion Cliffs area with someone who'd been leading camping tours in the desert for years.

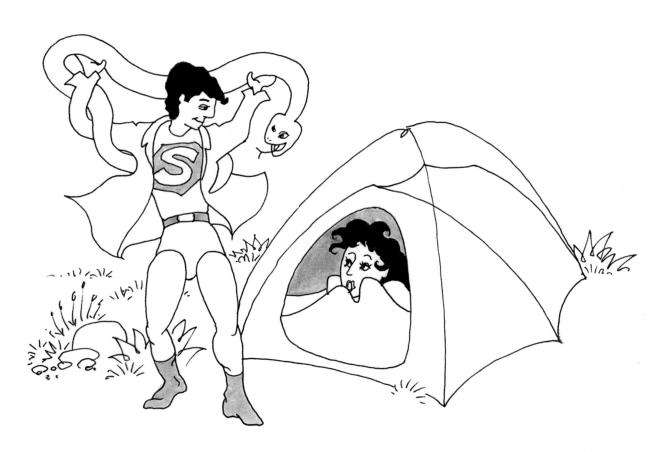

As he moved between a boulder and a bush, he suddenly exposed a snake in our path—and, much to my surprise, he jumped! So I figure if a snake can make a guy like that jump, the rest of us have nothing to be ashamed of.

Luckily, snakes tend to get out of the way when they sense people are around. But it's possible to run into them now and then, and it might be enough to panic you or your partner into doing something silly. If there are any dangerous snakes in the area where you'll be camping, it's a good idea to know how to recognize them, so you can avoid unnecessary anxiety every time a harmless snake crosses your path. In areas with lots of poisonous snakes, a snakebite kit is worth packing. I know it would make me feel better about my chances after a close encounter.

If you have a partner who is seriously afraid of snakes, you can be a real hero by checking their boots and sleeping bag to make sure there are no snakes lurking in there. By taking the lead on any hiking trails, you can also be the one to ensure that there are no killer serpents waiting to strike around the next bend.

Bugs

As I've mentioned, this one hits close to home. I still don't like them, but I've mostly recovered from my fear of bugs; at least they don't immediately make my pulse race anymore. I put annoying bugs into two categories: creepy-crawlies and biting bugs.

Creepy-crawlies are things like centipedes, beetles, grasshoppers, and other insects that don't actually pose any threat but do play on some people's irrational fears. If your partner is grossed out by bugs, don't just laugh it off. You won't be getting much loving from someone who's totally freaked out.

Keeping your tent door zipped up at all times will make it impossible for these bugs to get inside. Having a "safe" sleeping environment is a must if you're going to enjoy

camping (especially if you want to have sex in there), so if your partner is nervous, offer to go into the tent first and check for bugs. It might seem pointless to you, but it's a small effort to put someone you care about at ease. Once the inside of the tent is deemed safe, you'll have less trouble getting your partner's clothes off! The other place where a bug-hater might feel nervous is the outhouse, so offer to check that out first as well. You can even score extra points by standing guard outside the door.

Almost everyone who camps thinks that biting bugs are a big pain. Mosquitoes, black flies, deer flies, and other biters can turn a beautiful night in the wilderness into an itchy nightmare. I made the mistake of taking my boyfriend camping in Quebec during the worst part of black fly season. Thousands of them swarmed around us as soon as we got to the campsite. We had to put on our rain gear just to keep the flies from biting through our clothes. My poor boyfriend got massacred while we were putting up the tent. By the time we were done, his entire face was covered in blood. I'm lucky he didn't dump me right then and there.

There are a few different ways to deal with these bloodsuckers if someone is so bothered by them that he or she refuses to camp. The easiest solution is to avoid camping during the summer months. At other times of the year, most biting bugs are simply not around in large numbers. If you're willing to trade long days and warm weather for peace of mind, then a bit of creative scheduling is all you need to keep your partner happy.

If you can't avoid being around biting bugs, then the next best thing is to prevent them from biting. This means creating some kind of physical or chemical barrier to keep them away from you. Pack a good bug repellent to whip out as soon as you see the first mosquito of the day.

If you or your partner are not terribly happy about spraying deet all over your bodies, invest in bug-proof jackets, pants, and hats that are made of tight netting. It might

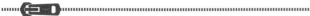

Driving
Me Buggy!

" I absolutely hate bugs. Can't stand them! Sitting outside for a barbeque during the summer drove me nuts if there were bugs around. I would get those citronella candles and completely surround myself with them. There was no way I was going camping with no house to run and hide inside. My husband, convinced that I would like it if I could just get over the bug thing, really wanted me to come on a camping trip with him. I told him the only way I would consider it was if he could actually guarantee I wouldn't get any mosquito bites. I figured that was impossible, so I'd never have to go camping.

My husband thought I was being a bit ridiculous, but he went out and bought me a "Don't Bug Me" jacket and pants and promised me that they would make me bug-proof. After trying it out in the backyard (and having my husband laugh his head off at me), I agreed to go camping with him. I have to admit that it wasn't as bad as I expected, and we still go camping at least once every summer. But I never go without my bug jacket! **"**

—DB

seem like an extreme way to deal with the problem, but if that's what it takes to make someone feel safe from biting bugs, then it's worth taking some extra stuff along. On the plus side, if you manage to keep the bugs out of your tent, you can happily strip away your bug-proof clothing once inside.

Getting Lost

I'm the first to admit that I have a terrible sense of direction. Whenever I'm leading a hike, I begin by telling the other hikers, "If you think I'm going the wrong way, speak up. I probably am!" So I've learned to use marked trails as much as possible and to stop often and check the map. Even so, I took one woman on a hike in a river valley just outside of Toronto, and we managed to get so caught up in our conversation that we ended up walking in a complete circle before I realized we'd taken a wrong turn. And that was just in the suburbs! So far, I've never been so badly lost that I couldn't make my way back to the right trail. But I do harbor a secret fear that one day I'll be in the middle of the woods with no idea where I am.

If you aren't comfortable in the bush, the fear of getting lost and wandering aimlessly until all hope fades can be pretty overwhelming. It's something that can happen to even the most experienced campers, so you always have to be ready in case it happens to you. A change in conditions, an un-crossable river, or a washed-out trail can send you off course. But there are ways to build up a beginner's confidence both before and during your trip.

Even if one of you is comfortable making your way through unmarked wilderness or finding a new shortcut, don't expect your partner to share your enthusiasm for cross-country exploration right away. For at least the first few trips you do together, stick to marked trails or simple canoe or kayak routes so your partner can see that you are staying on the right track. Sometimes all it takes to put someone's mind at ease is the reassurance of seeing a blaze or a signpost. Show your partner on the map exactly where you are, and do it more often than you think you should—every five or 10 minutes is a good idea if your partner is worried about it.

If you're extremely nervous about getting lost, even on a marked trail, plan your first trip along a heavily used route. Running into other people on a regular basis will be reassuring and keep you or your partner from thinking that you could be stranded alone in the woods. You'll have to sacrifice some of the privacy you'd find on less popular trails, but until you're comfortable, you aren't likely to enjoy the privacy much anyway. Campers are a friendly bunch, so if you run into people coming from the opposite way, you can ask them about the terrain up ahead, and how far you are from your destination.

Maps are important on any camping trip. Before the trip, spread out the map on a table and look over your route and where you'll be stopping each night if you aren't returning to a base camp. Pay attention to landmarks like rivers, lakes, and bridges that will be recognizable as you pass them on your trip. If you get familiar with the route before you're on it, you won't feel as powerless and dependent on your more experienced partner.

Personally, I like to use this kind of landmark technique to keep me motivated on a long walk. I'll check out the map for points that will be easy to recognize, like a footbridge we have to cross. Then when we get there, I know exactly how far along the route we've gone, and how much is left to go. It's also a good way to know if I've somehow taken the wrong trail. If I'm supposed to cross a bridge after 1 mile, and two hours later I still haven't crossed it, it's time to think about where I might have made a wrong turn. Bodies of water are the easiest to spot, along with buildings (like huts, for instance), cliffs, and ridges. Remember that a small stream marked on a map may not be there during a dry spell, or a new stream that's not marked on the map may appear after a storm. Never rely on just one landmark, but on the various ones you pass along the whole route.

Better still, learn how to use a compass and map to find your own way. Navigating and orienteering skills are very empowering and build confidence. If you've got the time before you head out, take a navigation course. Even if your partner is willing to help you, sometimes a proper teacher makes a big difference in picking up new knowledge. Knowledge is power, and power will give you the confidence to face the wilderness. If you want to take things a step further, it is now quite feasible to carry your very own GPS (global-positioning system) receiver on your camping trips. They are small, lightweight, and can tell you precisely where you are.

Another thing to do before you leave is tell someone where you are going and when you expect to be back. If there is someone back in civilization waiting to call out the troops if you don't show up when you're supposed to, it will add an extra level of assurance.

Cold

If you've never slept outside, you're probably expecting to get cold on your camping trip. After all, we live in houses for a good reason. My boyfriend, Gerhard, is always cold. He'll wear two fleece jackets inside the house. So it may seem kind of surprising that he likes going camping, even when it's not summer. Giving up the comfort of a warm bed is something that makes a lot of people shy away from camping. But as Gerhard knows, there's just no reason to be cold on a camping trip if you take the right stuff with you.

With proper clothing, a good sleeping bag, and a tent, you'll be in for a cozy night in almost any conditions. (Of course, if you're new to camping, you may want to avoid doing your first trip in the middle of winter, just to be safe.) If you know that you get cold easily, remember to

It's in the Bag

66 My only memory of camping out as a kid was shivering all night in my sleeping bag and wishing I was home. So when I spent the first night in the down sleeping bag I borrowed from my friend, I was wearing about ten layers of clothing. It took about five minutes for me to start sweating buckets and stripping off layers of fleece. My girlfriend thought I was a complete nutcase. I guess I must have looked like one. I wonder what my childhood sleeping bag was made of—old bed sheets, maybe? 99

—RS

pack extra layers. Dry socks, warm gloves, and a wool or fleece hat can turn a chilly night into a perfect opportunity to cuddle. And don't hold back on the cuddling! It will not only keep you both warm, but also distract you from the fact that it's cold outside.

If you share your sleeping bags, you can benefit from the extra warmth of your partner's body heat. There are a number of double-size sleeping bags available. But most brands' single bags can be zipped together into a double as well, if you buy one left-opening and one right-opening bag. You can even combine different models and/or brands into one "interspecies" bag if the zippers are the same size and the bags are roughly the same shape and length. Whatever brand you go with, check at the store to make sure that the bags will "mate." And then be prepared for a little mating of your own! A double bag makes it much easier to get intimate without getting cold at the same time. So if you're hoping to have a romantic night even though the temperature has dropped, the double bag is ideal. Before you know it, you'll both be complaining about how hot it is in there.

In areas that allow it, a campfire can be a romantic way to stay warm after sundown without having to hide inside your tent right away. Sitting beside a crackling fire is one of my favorite things about camping, especially if I get to snuggle with my man. It's like a candlelight dinner a hundred times over. The smell of the wood smoke permeates my camping clothes and acts as a reminder of the romantic night by the fire for the rest of the trip. As an added bonus, the smoke helps to keep bugs away. It's not always possible or practical to light a fire, but if the campsite has a fire pit and there's no ban in place, it's a great way to spend the evening together. Just don't go cutting down trees to get fuel.

If you're afraid that camping will entail spending the night shivering away, pack a few marshmallows and look forward to sitting by a cozy fire toasting them together. Then snuggle into your warm sleeping bags and make a real effort to heat things up in your tent.

Great Balls of Fire!

66 When I met my future husband, I made it very clear that I was not an "outdoorsy" kind of person. I like to be warm, dry, and comfortable, thank you very much. But as things got more and more serious between us, he started trying to subtly suggest that if I gave it a try, I might just enjoy myself. It took an awful lot of convincing, but by the time we got married, I was willing to give it a shot.

On our very first camping trip together, it rained all day. My husband tried to console me by making a nice campfire, but, of course, the wood was all wet and he couldn't get it to light. He was so determined to show me he could light a fire that he poured lighter fluid all over the thing, and when he threw in the match, it went up like a big fireball and nearly burned his eyebrows off! And then it went out again anyway.

Lucky for him, the sun came out the next day, and the rest of our trip was really nice. Otherwise, that might have been the end of camping for me. But now I actually have learned to love the outdoors, and while I still prefer to sleep in my bed, I can give it up now and then. 99

--TS

Rain

It's a fact of life that if you go camping, you will eventually encounter some rainy weather. You might as well be ready for it. Try out your rain gear on a stormy day at home to make sure that it does keep the water out. Knowing that you have the right gear will help you to relax on your trip.

A little rain might not be so bad if you have ways to pass the time. Pack a deck of cards and a couple of

Working Up
to a Proposal

Greg and I were on a ski trip in the Italian Alps. Unfortunately, there was no fresh snow and it was incredibly foggy every day, but we were in the Alps, so we weren't complaining. In the evenings, we joined our friends for wonderful family meals.

One day, the sun finally came out, so Greg and I decided to take a drive to a different ski area, Claviere.

When Greg plays, he likes do things a more "interesting" way. With snowboarding, this means hiking to reach good powder. Although I am often willing to come along, I tend to be lazy and lethargic after lunch. Needless to say, when Greg picked up his board and started hiking out to a ridge, I wasn't thrilled. In fact, I was feeling quite nauseated hiking after the meal. *Can't we, for once, take it a bit easy?* I thought. I might even admit to being a bit whiny. Greg was urging me on. When he stopped so I could sit and rest, I thought, *Wow, I got off easy.*

It was beautiful: We were sitting on a knife-edge ridge surrounded by snow-covered peaks. In the distant valley, we could see the alpine towns. This is my memory of what happened next (Greg has a somewhat different version):

Greg: "Is this pretty?"

Me: "Yes."

Greg: "Is it romantic?"

Me: "Yes."

Greg: "No, really, I mean, is it *really* romantic?"

Well, I could hardly think because my heart started beating really fast as I said, "*Yessss......*"

Then Greg got down on his knees in the snow and pulled out a box wrapped in a Borders coupon. I don't remember the entire conversation clearly from that point on because I was too busy crying. I think he said he got me a 25-percent-off Borders coupon, and I said I always wanted that. Underneath was a little blue box with a ring inside. He proposed, and I said yes.

We sat there for a while. I was very excited that no one else knew our little secret, except for the skiers hanging out on the hut's deck. We decide to go down, and I had an awesome afternoon scoring freshies in the trees.

On the way back, we stopped by the town of Cesana to walk around. At this point, I no longer wanted to keep the secret. I wanted to tell someone, anyone. We went to a wine bar and ordered two glasses of Barolo. I asked Greg if I could tell our waitress. He said sure, probably wondering how I would accomplish that. Well, in the international language of women, I pointed to my ring and said, "Oggi," which means "today" in Italian. Of course, she understood. And I discovered the way to get a free plate of appetizers: She brought us over a plate of bread, prosciutto, and cheese. Maybe we should try that more often...

—*Wanda Gonzalez*

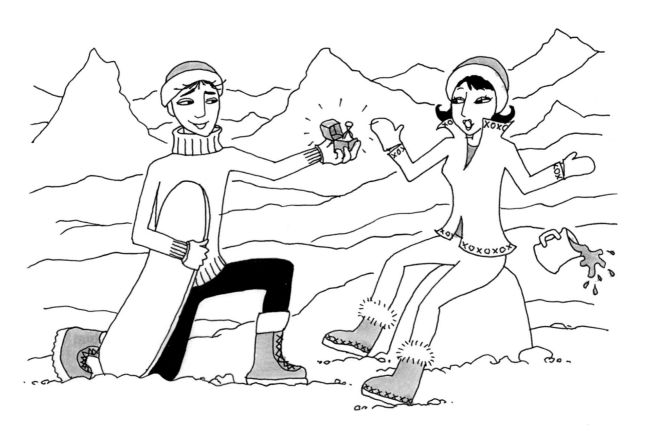

magazines, and bring an extra tarp and ropes for some shelter outside of the tent. Of course, a rainy night (or day) is a perfect excuse to hide in your tent for a little extra snuggling and sex. Might as well stay warm!

Ease Into It

Yes, it's possible to have too much of a good thing, especially your first time out. Don't get carried away with your enthusiasm for showing your partner all of the great stuff you can do on a camping trip. Start slow, start small, and gradually make your camping trips more challenging as your partner gets more comfortable. My friend Maria is a beginner camper, but she is willing to try new things because she trusts her boyfriend to understand where her comfort level is. "I feel I can trust him 100 percent with the plans and details of the trip that I may be more unsure of," she says. "I can trust his judgment, trust his sense of what is a challenge versus what is dangerous, and I can trust that he takes my abilities into account."

Let's look at some ways to make those first few trips easier for someone who's still not too sure about all of this outdoorsy stuff, and build their trust to the point where they're willing to try more challenging outings.

Start at Home

If you've got a partner who is terrified of camping, try "practicing" at home first. If you have a yard, set up your tent there and spend a night in it together. Your partner will get a chance to see how warm and comfortable it can be, without ever being too far from a real bed. It will also give you a heads up on any extra comforts that your partner might need on a trip, like a travel pillow or a set of earplugs. Do it right by wearing the clothes you would bring with you on a camping trip.

You can also try out some of your camping meals at home before you go. If your secret recipe for tuna pasta supreme makes your partner gag, it's better to find out before it's the only thing you've got.

The More the Merrier

66 My husband kept saying he wanted me to come mountain biking with him, because it would be so much fun if we could do it together. So finally I said OK, I'd give it a try. But then as soon as we were on the trail, he just took off and left me (literally, might I add) in his dust. I wasn't really sure where the trail went, or if it branched off anywhere.

By the time I caught up with him, he had been waiting for 15 minutes, and he was ready to take off as soon as he saw I was OK. So I didn't rest at all, and this pretty much kept happening all day. As soon as I caught up, he'd take off again. At the end of the day I said, "If that's your idea of spending the day together, you might as well go by yourself."

We eventually found a compromise. We go biking with a group so he can take off with the fast people, and I can follow along with the slower ones and not be left alone. 99

–HU

And be sure to try out some of the sexy suggestions in Chapter 5—you may find your partner is converted into an enthusiastic camper on the spot!

Bring the Car

Car camping can be an excellent way to introduce someone to the outdoors and get a new camper comfortable before trying to go into a park interior. Even if you are an experienced backcountry camper, take your partner on a car-camping trip the first couple of times. Having a vehicle nearby makes people feel safe, since you can always make a quick escape back to civilization. Car camping also gives you the option of bringing along more comforts

Sexy Tent Games for a Rainy Day

If the weather's bad, there's no need to pack up your trip. Take the opportunity to hole up in your tent for a little romance. If you need help getting started, try one of my favorite games.

STRIP POKER:

Try the classic version or substitute your favorite card game. If you don't have cards, try Strip 20 Questions. Pick a famous person to be (maybe someone naughty like Madonna or the Marquis de Sade), and let your partner guess who you are by asking questions with yes or no answers. For every question they need to ask, your partner loses an article of clothing. Chances are, you'll never get to 20!

TEQUILA PIGS:

These little plastic piggies were designed as a drinking game, but you can bring along your own rules. When you throw the pig down, how it lands determines what you have to do. Snout down, remove a piece of clothing. Bum down, remove a piece of your partner's clothing. Lying on one side, kiss an exposed part of your partner. Standing up, your partner has to perform the sexual act of your choice (time limits may apply). It's even more fun than tequila, and you won't get a hangover!

STORY TIME:

Take turns telling a sexy tale, with each person adding the next sentence. You can set the scene by making your story take place on a camping trip. Start of with something like:

"Once upon a time, a handsome, young man (or beautiful, young woman) was walking through the woods." Then the next person continues: "Suddenly, he saw something in the river ahead of him—someone bathing naked." Well, you can see where this is going, but let your imaginations run free.

STRIP BATTLESHIP:

You'll need to bring the travel version of this game along. Each time one of you sinks an opponent's ship, the defeated player will have to give up an article of clothing. Fire at will, and prepare the torpedoes for action.

PLAYING DOCTOR:

When was the last time you were thoroughly examined?

I NEVER!:

Tell each other the hottest things you've never done but want to try. Perhaps you've never given an erotic massage, or gone outside naked in the rain.

TRUTH OR DARE:

Time to find out about each other's secret side. Has your partner every had fantasies about a friend? Have you ever slept with someone you had no interest in seeing again? Tell the truth!

69 SHOWDOWN:

Who can experience oral sex longer before reaching orgasm? There are no real losers in this game!

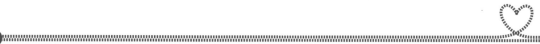

of home since you don't have as many limits on size and weight. And if things get really bad weather-wise, you can always hide in the car and turn the heat on—or even retreat to the nearest motel.

Keep It Short

Save those plans for the transcontinental hike for a little later. To begin, go away for a weekend trip. One night in the woods together will get your partner used to sleeping in a tent, cooking meals outside, and facing any lingering fears. What it won't do is leave your partner exhausted, filthy, and desperate for civilization. Nobody will have to worry about getting lost on a long, backcountry trail or river system, miles away from anywhere. The trip also will be easier to plan and pack for than a longer expedition.

A simple car-camping trip to a park with scenic dayhikes can be a great introduction to camping. Dayhikes with a small pack are less daunting than backpacking with everything you need to set up camp. Likewise, paddling around a lake and returning to a base camp is far easier than loading up a canoe or kayak with all of your belongings and carrying them over portages, while still offering a bit of the scenery you'd see during a paddling trip.

Bring Backup

If your partner has a lot of doubts about being able to hack it with only you to rely on, bring along more people. (This may seem counter to the idea of a romantic weekend, but remember, you can always pitch your tent in a secluded spot.) There is strength in numbers, and your partner may feel safer if you're not the only one around to help in an emergency. It also takes some of the pressure off of you, since you'll have more experienced help around. If you know another couple who like camping, invite them along for a weekend. This can be particularly helpful for women first-timers, who may feel much more comfortable with another woman around

to ask for advice. After all, no man has to squat in the bush to pee!

Spoil Your Partner

Bring things along that you know will put your partner at ease, even if those items aren't exactly necessary for camping. Have his or her favorite chocolate bar or cookies as a treat, or a little wine or sherry. If you're car camping, you can even bring a cooler of beer. Anything that will give an emotional boost to your partner, without being completely inappropriate, would be a good idea to take along.

For Doug, getting his wife out on her first canoe trip involved a lot of coercion. "My wife was very reluctant to camp—she figured it would be a painful experience with nothing but getting wet, dirty, and cold," he says. "In the middle of the winter, we were visiting with friends, and the discussion turned to doing a canoe weekend together as families. My wife agreed, thinking it would never happen."

When they actually started planning the trip, she wanted to back out. She tried thinking of creative excuses to tell the other couple why they couldn't do it. But her husband knew if he could just get her to see the beautiful surroundings, she'd really enjoy herself. It called for extreme measures.

"I talked her into going based on me doing everything: All the packing, portaging, setting up camp, cooking, cleaning the dishes—*and* she got to bring a lawn chair," he says. "As it turned out, she fell in love with it. She has insisted on going every summer since."

A good first impression made all the difference for Doug and his wife. If you're trying to find ways to convince your partner, think of all the little details that will make the trip more comfortable. Sometimes it's as simple as an inflatable pillow to make sleeping more comfortable, or a blindfold to keep the sunrise from waking him or her up. For some people, it's worth packing real cream to put in the morning coffee, or real coffee instead of instant. Try to identify a few of these things that will make the first few times easier for your partner, and make sure you have them handy.

You can also spoil your partner by lavishing extra attention on him or her. Whisper sweet nothings, steal kisses, give a massage, and make it clear that you are willing to do whatever it takes to make this experience a good one.

Time Your Trip

It may seem kind of obvious, but if your partner hates mosquitoes, don't go on your first trip when it's mosquito season. If you have pollen allergies, don't go camping when flowers are pollinating. Planning your first camping experiences to avoid the conditions that would upset you or your partner is the easiest way to make the most of the positive stuff and downplay the negative.

The weatherman should be part of your trip planning, too. If you were hoping to go away for the weekend and the weather forecast says there's going to be constant rain or a violent storm, it may be worth putting your trip on hold. If your partner's first experience is really awful, it will be hard to convince him or her to give it another try. Of course, bad weather is eventually going to come up on a camping trip, but if you can avoid the extremes to begin with, things will probably go much more smoothly. Ross Morton, who has worked with Outward Bound for seven years, says the most important thing in introducing a new camper to the wilderness is timing. "I've had relationships with people who weren't outdoorsy," he says. "If you want to take someone up a mountain, you wait for a beautiful, sunny day to do it."

Pick Your Spot

Going to the right place can be just as important to the first camping experience as the right timing. Try to find a place that will have gorgeous scenery that is also within your partner's comfort zone. Don't plan to climb a

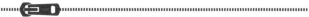

Love = Caffeine

❝ My wife is not a morning person at all. Whenever we went camping, she refused to get out of her sleeping bag in the morning, and it would take an hour to get her up. Then she'd be grumpy for the whole time we broke down the campsite. I tried waking her gently, but that didn't work. I tried to get her excited about what we had planned for the day, but she never seemed to care about that, either. I was at a loss.

One day, I was up a little earlier than usual, so I went outside and made coffee. I poured a cup for her, complete with cream and sugar, and brought it into the tent. I woke her up and handed her the coffee without her having to leave the warmth of her sleeping bag. After that, she was chipper for the rest of the day. So now that's our morning routine—coffee in bed for my honey. The things we do for love! ❞

—BV

huge mountain or shoot Class V rapids on your first trip together. Make it achievable and enjoyable. You can work your way up to Mt. Everest later.

If you have been camping for a while, it's a good idea to take your beginner partner somewhere you've already been. That way, you'll know what to expect, and you can make sure your partner is prepared for what's coming up next. If you're considering your first camping trip, be realistic about your abilities. You might want to see some great place your partner has raved about, but if it's a five-day hike to get there, don't suggest it for your first trip. Keep your plans in line with your experience.

Involve the Beginner

Even if you are used to doing everything yourself, make sure you get your partner to help you set up the tent, prepare dinner, and make camp comfortable. Nothing makes you feel quite as useless as standing around watching someone else set up the entire campsite while you have no idea what to do with yourself. Start with simple stuff like setting up the sleeping pads and bags inside the tent. My boyfriend has his special way of tying the tent down with ropes, so I make myself useful by gathering rocks for him to use to hold the ropes down if there aren't enough trees around. (It's the most useful thing I can do, because heaven knows I'll never remember how to tie his special knot!)

By handing over a few new tasks every time you camp together, you involve your beginner and, little by little, you will teach him or her how to be a camper. Make sure you explain why things are done the way they are, rather than just bossing your partner around. Feeling useless is bad, but feeling like a slave is worse. Beginners, ask lots of questions if you don't understand why your partner is doing something a particular way. It could be important for safety–or it could just be a personal preference. The sooner the beginner learns how to do camping tasks, the sooner the experienced one can stop doing them all, and the more time the two of you will get to spend on the fun activities, like christening the tent.

Offer Lots of Encouragement

If you're not used to it, carrying a backpack or paddling all day is a hell of a lot of work! Keep this in mind and remember to stop and see how your partner is doing now and then, and offer some encouragement. Tell your partner how far you have already gone, and how close you are to your next stop. Keep it positive, and stop for extra hugs and kisses along the way. Your partner wants to feel appreciated, and to know that you're glad he or she is with you. Don't take this for granted, but say it out loud and say it often: "I'm so happy that you agreed to try this." "I'm so glad you're here with me to see this." With luck, by the end of the trip, your partner will be saying it right back to you.

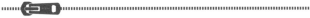

Definitely Not *the Beginner's Route*

❝ We had our hearts set on camping next to this creek, but it was more than 100 feet below us, deep within a canyon that seemed inaccessible. Finally, we found a wash that led into the canyon. Once we climbed down the first 10 feet of the wash, we had to cut our switchback down the steep walls of the canyon to get to the cliff. From there, it was a sheer, 10-foot drop to a sandstone shelf on which we planned to camp. Hiking down the switchback was frightening because the dirt was loose; one wrong step, and I would have fallen over the edge of a 75-foot cliff. I decided to take that switchback on my butt because it was safer. Then, in order for us to get to the bottom of the cliff, we had to lower our backpacks by rope and rock climb down an alcove in the cliff.

The next morning after breakfast, we packed up camp and headed out of the canyon. First, we had to lift the backpacks up the cliff by rope. Then we had to climb back up the switchback to the wash. I did so on all fours because the dirt was too loose for me, and I dropped my hiking stick. It landed next to the river. Scared and angry, I stood in the wash and tried to catch my breath. John asked me if I was okay; I shook my head. He asked me if I wanted him to get my hiking stick out of the canyon; I nodded. By the time he returned with the stick, I had finally recovered from my fright, and I hugged and kissed him, happy to be alive. ❞

—*Heather Verley*

Usually, the hardest part of converting someone into a camper is getting them out on that first trip. After that, you shouldn't have any trouble making plans for other camping trips. Just remember the old cliché (because it's actually true in this case), you never get a second chance to make a first impression.

Ready for Action

Once you're both feeling comfortable with the camping basics, you can let your sense of romance and adventure start to roam free. By breaking out of your routine, your sex life can take new directions you may not have considered before. Ever had a Tarzan fantasy? Tarzan can hide up in the treetops, observing the human female that has wandered unknowingly into his territory. The first he has ever seen! He can't communicate with her in the usual way, never having learned to speak. Jane is afraid but intrigued by the rugged stranger. Who is this wild man? What is he going to do to me? Tarzan curiously compares her body to his own, feeling his way around her. He must remove her clothing to see what she is hiding beneath it. His instincts begin to take over, and he soon realizes what these new feelings are telling him to do. He backs her up against a tree and makes love to her, discovering the sex act for the very first time.

You've got to admit, it's a far cry from the usual routine. The possibilities are endless if you've got an active imagination. How about Han Solo and Princess Leia celebrating among the Ewoks? Or you could be two contestants on *Survivor,* trying to escape from the prying eyes of the cameras to have a private night together. This is your chance to get out of the bedroom and shake things up!

Is your partner convinced yet? Read on to start making plans for your first (or next) hot trip into the wilderness. Once the two of you bring a passion for the outdoors into your relationship, there's no limit to where you take it.

Chapter 2:

PLANNING A TRIP

that Won't End Your Relationship

I love my boyfriend. I love camping. So how is it that in the middle of a camping trip with Gerhard, I found myself so miserable that I was in tears? Let me tell you, he was pretty anxious to find out the answer to that question, too.

After a long day of driving out to the campground in heavy rain and fog, it was pouring rain when we arrived. All through the process of trying to pitch the tent and make dinner in a downpour, he kept bossing me around, telling me how to do every last little thing. After the stress of the drive, and his back-seat driving (from the front seat), it was more than I could take. I was cold, wet, frustrated, and starting to question our entire relationship. Clearly, Gerhard didn't think much of me if he couldn't leave me to do the least little task my own way. How could I have a fulfilling relationship with someone who thought I was a moron?

When he cornered me and asked what was wrong, he was more than a little surprised to find out what was going on in my head. It turns out he had no idea I was so bothered by how much he was trying to "help." I realized then that he couldn't possibly have known, because I never said a word about it until I burst into tears. Somehow, I was counting on him to read my mind, something we girls do more often than we like to admit. Gerhard agreed to back off and let me do my own thing more.

By the next day, the sun came out, and I felt like an idiot for thinking that our whole relationship was falling apart because I had a bad day. But when it comes to camping, it's easy to blow things out of proportion.

Ross Morton of Outward Bound agrees that things can get more tense when conditions are not what you'd hoped. "The wilderness experience can make or break relationships," he says. "It's an amazing thing to share moments in the bush. But it can be a challenge when you're stuck on a mountain for three days in the rain."

Author Kathleen Meyer sees conflict on a camping trip as a kind of litmus test for the whole relationship. "If

one of the couple is fearful of experiencing new things, or feeling uncomfortable with sleeping on the ground or whatever, I think if there are other parts of your relationship that aren't solid, it ignites those parts," she says.

On the other hand, Meyer says, the problems you face can also help strengthen your bond. "If your outdoor excursion with your partner is at all arduous, and your relationship should survive it, then that bond you create out there can translate into home life and helping you balance things," she says. "It's a good way to find out if you're going to last with somebody. It's better to find out sooner than later!"

Anytime two people are in each other's company 24 hours a day, there is a pretty good chance that they'll get on one another's nerves and start to fight, even if they love each other. Out in the middle of the wilderness with nobody else around, this could be a real problem—and not just at the time; the effects can be felt long after. You can get into a fight about all kinds of things on camping trips: getting lost, forgetting gear at home, where to go, how long to stay, how fast to travel, what to eat. But there's no need to let this stuff get in the way of having a great trip together, and staying in love with each other. After all, spending time outside together puts you in new and challenging situations, which give you an opportunity to discover something new to admire about each other. A lot of the arguments that come up can be avoided by planning well.

The Destination vs. the Journey

One of the main differences in the way people envision their camping trips is that some of us prefer to plan for a specific destination, like reaching the top of a mountain or completing a trail, and other people are all about the journey. They're more likely to be looking for wildlife or stopping to admire the view. If one of you is destination-oriented and the other is not, it might be tough to figure out how you're both going to get what you want. It's time for a bit of planning and compromise. Make sure you have plenty of time to achieve the goals that mean a lot to the destination person, whether it's getting to the mouth of a river or the top of a mountain. If you know you can easily make it in the time you've allowed, you're less likely to feel the need to rush onward all of the time, which the stop-and-smell-the-flowers person will appreciate.

Susan and her husband suffered from this problem for some time before arriving at a simple solution. "My husband is very competitive," Susan says. "He works in sales, and he's always excited when he lands a tough customer or he blows his quota out of the water. He's the kind of guy who has to buy every new gadget before any of his friends have one."

When it comes to camping, Susan's husband is the same way, which drives Susan, who likes to take it easy, absolutely crazy. When he came home with a wrist-top GPS, Susan shook her head, imagining how this new gizmo would feed her husband's minute-by-minute obsession with how far they could go on their outings. "He wants to do everything farther and faster than normal," she explains. "So if a hike was supposed to take six hours, and we did it in five hours, it was like we 'won' somehow."

Susan felt guilty on their trips, as if she were holding him back. One day, she couldn't handle it anymore, and she told her husband she never wanted to go camping with him again. "When he asked why, I couldn't believe it!" she says. "It turned out he had no idea that I didn't share his enthusiasm for 'challenging' ourselves."

Then he asked her why she had never said anything before. "I guess I was just trying to keep him happy, at my own expense," she says. "Now we plan our trips to alternate one easy day for each 'challenging' day, and I actually enjoy myself—at least half the time."

Outward Bound's Ross Morton acknowledges that Susan's story is not that unusual. "Guys tend to want to get on with it," he says. "They want to just throw on their packs and get moving. Women tend to be more cautious. They want to talk first and make sure they understand (the

plan)." It's as if our camping lives mirror our sex lives. Typically, men want to get straight into the action, while women are more willing to relax into things if they get to talk about it first and have some "pre-adventure" foreplay.

For some campers, the challenge of accomplishing their goals in record time is half the fun. If you're one of these people, allowing extra time to enjoy the scenery is just annoying. If you have tough goals that your partner doesn't share, it may be worth saving them for another trip with a friend who shares the same goal. It's never a good idea to force your partner to do something that he or she thinks is too difficult or dangerous. You'll just end up with a tired, crabby, and potentially scared-to-death partner on your hands. And who do you think is going to get the blame?

Make some time to talk about your route before the trip, so that you can both point out what's important to you. One of you might be dying to do some climbing on a well-known rock face, and the other might want to spend some time at a spot that's perfect for seeing rare birds. Plan it so that you both get to do the things that are most important to you, even if you think bird-watching is stupid and boring, or that rock climbing is a foolish risk of life. That way each of you can take a turn at compromising, and each of you comes away from the trip having seen or done what you most wanted to see or do.

Couples therapist Esther Perel says that there are times, both in our sex lives and in our hobbies, when we're better off keeping our more extreme behaviors for our own time if they aren't shared by our partners. "If you're into something, before you share it, you have to ask yourself if there's a certain fit," she says. "Will the other person be open to it? Will they be threatened or turned off by it?"

When it comes to playing together, the lines can blur between what happens during the day and how you feel about each other later on. So if your partner feels like you've been making unreasonable demands on him or her all day, chances are you're not going to find them very anxious to please you that night. Sometimes it may be best if your life partner isn't always your sports partner.

Jaime and her partner Harris are a bit of an unusual couple. Even though they've been together for eight years, they each live in their own homes in different suburbs. "We've both been married before, and we think this works better for us—the independence of being single combined with the companionship of having a partner," explains Jaime. So it's a bit of a surprise that they get along so well on camping holidays, where they're together 24/7 for as long as four weeks. It's a lot of time to spend together without a break, especially for two people who don't have all of the same interests.

How do they do it? Jaime says they usually make separate lists of things they'd like to see or do, and then they compare the lists and make a rough itinerary. "I know that he's a stronger backpacker than I am (Harris used to do some mountaineering), so if he really wants to do a climb somewhere, we'll just plan it so that I have a rest day while he goes on his own," she says. Sometimes recognizing that you don't have to do everything together is the best approach. "I'm happy to have a day of solitude and do some gentle walks on my own, while he gets to reach the summits he likes so much," Jaime says. "So both of our needs are met."

For Dimitri and his wife, camping together has been a lesson in compromise. "It's made us more aware of each other's likes and dislikes, strengths and weaknesses," he says. "It's made us more tolerant toward each other. It's made us realize the joy of doing and sharing things together." Not only are these important qualities when they're in the woods, but he also finds that they can cope better with tough situations in their day-to-day life. If you've experienced getting lost in the woods, it's not going to seem like such a big deal if you get lost driving in a new city. If you've learned to survive in a tent, there's nothing scary about a power blackout.

Some compromises may be less of a choice and more of a necessity. Are you both at the same level of fitness? Can your partner keep up with your ambitious plans? Can you both get the same amount of time off work for the trip? Do you both have the right gear for the activities you are planning? Being physically ready and properly geared up for a trip is a key part of your planning. Halfway up a mountain is a bad time to figure out that one of you isn't fit enough to go on.

Incorporate What You Love to Do

You and your partner probably each have your own hobbies at home. It's important for the health of your relationship to give one another the space to take part in those interests, separately if necessary. The activities you include in your camping trips are no different. Photography, bird-watching, rock climbing, sketching, and swimming are just a few of the things that people pursue to make their camping trips more interesting. These activities are a big part of the appeal of camping, and if you're denied the chance to do them, it can seem like the whole trip was a waste of time. Ideally, you'll still enjoy everything else you're doing, like spending time with your partner and getting away from the city for a while. But for some people, a trip where they don't get to do their favorite thing isn't much fun.

If you're lucky enough to have the same hobbies as your partner, you're all set. But if you want to stop and sketch, and your partner is left sitting around waiting for you, it can lead to unnecessary tension. You end up feeling guilty every time you indulge in your hobby, and your partner gets bored and impatient. For instance, I like to take pictures, while my boyfriend prefers to take naps. So I tend to make frequent stops along our route whenever I see anything I want to photograph, while he would rather carry on through and get to our destination early enough to fit in an afternoon snooze. It takes some compromise for us both to get what we want. But I'll try to limit my photo stops to the most breathtaking vistas

Getting to Know
the Real You

As a lifelong outdoorswoman, I have always been attracted to guys who share one of my outdoor interests. Not only is it great to share an activity I love with a guy I'm attracted to, it's also a good way to get to know the guy. When you're in a challenging environment, it's tough to "act," which means that if I still like the guy after we head outside together, chances are it's the real thing. The corollary to this is that I can also find out quickly whether the guy is a dud.

Several years ago, I was dating a guy I met at the climbing gym who wanted to take me traditional climbing—the kind of rock climbing where you place your own gear in the rock and scale the cliffs all on your own power. I was a fairly novice climber and had climbed outside only a handful of times, and only on single-pitch, bolted routes, so I was both nervous and excited to try "trad" climbing.

I felt confident that my new boyfriend was a capable climber, so I put my fears aside and joined him and two of his friends on a climbing trip to Red Rocks, outside of Las Vegas. Our road trip down from the San Francisco Bay Area was long. The car broke down, and even though I was worried it wouldn't get us to Vegas and back, my boyfriend insisted we keep going. That was my first sign that something wasn't right.

That night, we camped in Red Rocks and woke early for the climb. My boyfriend led the route, and when we got to the first anchor, I realized I should have talked to him about my concerns before we started climbing. I had no idea what I would do if he fell or got hurt, since my experience was limited to the comparatively safe gym environment. But instead of talking to him about my fear midway through our climb, I clenched my teeth and continued to belay for him.

As it turned out, the climb was fine, and I started to relax when our two friends, AR and JS, caught up to us at a ledge, where we took a break to eat. Once we reached the top and started our long walk to the car, my boyfriend announced that he was going to run back. I'm not sure why he was in such a hurry, but I had a nice chat with AR on the walk back, and I realized I didn't mind my boyfriend's absence.

The next day, we climbed some more, and on the third day, AR and I had to fly back early to return to work, while my boyfriend and JS stayed on to climb for another day. On that day, they had an epic: On their rappel down the cliff, they encountered a pair of climbers whose rope had gotten stuck. As they traversed to retrieve it, one of the climbers fell right near JS, who initially thought the climber had fallen to his death. Fortunately, he suffered only a broken ankle, but JS was so shaken by the sight of him falling that she clung to the anchor point to regain her composure.

When they finally got down from the climb, it was 1 or 2 in the morning, and my boyfriend and JS were so full of adrenaline that they decided to make the long drive home. When he told me the story later that night, he complained to me about JS holding onto the anchors. Recalling my own fear and inclination to grab the anchor after my first pitch, I told him I would have done the same thing.

Then he lost it. He started telling me I was irrational and that holding the anchors was stupid, and he finally concluded that he would never be able to climb with me again. We had been out plenty of times, but it wasn't until we had an outdoor challenge together that I saw his true colors, and we broke up that night.

The happy ending to this story is that I also saw the true colors of another guy on that trip, and AR and I have been together ever since. He is my favorite partner for climbing and skiing and all of life's challenges.

—ED

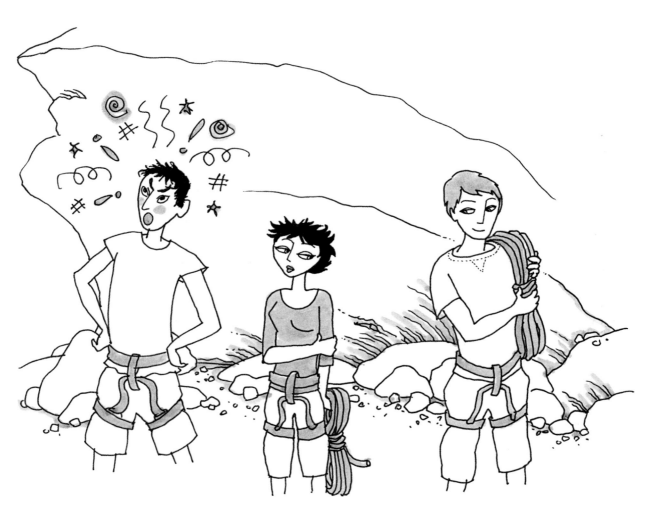

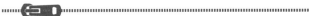

Creating a *Sketchy Memory*

" I have a little sketching kit that I bring along on every camping trip. It has my pencils and sharpeners and paper. To me, it's like a history of my outdoor experiences. I'll write little notes on the bottom saying where I was, and what time of year—maybe even a note on what colors things were. But it's mostly my impressions of the places we've been, and I keep them all in a box at home. My husband doesn't sketch, so I do it while he has a little rest. He's very big on scheduling sleeping times at least once per day while we're camping. It all works out well for us, except that I don't end up getting as many naps! **"**

—HT

(or fit them in when we've already stopped for a break) and then use the time while he's napping to wander around playing shutterbug.

Sometimes even having the same hobby can pose challenges. Lana and her husband both like to take pictures, so they're always fighting over the camera. "Not serious fighting, of course," Lana explains. "But we did have to go buy an extra memory card, because on longer trips we'd actually fill up our camera's memory, and neither of us ever wanted to delete any of our beautiful pictures." Lana's solution to their camera woes was simple: "Actually, my husband doesn't know this, but I'm getting him his own camera for his birthday so I can stop sharing mine."

Try to find some way to incorporate what you both like to do into the trip. If you're going to stop and sketch, plan to do it somewhere with a side trail for your partner to explore, or on a beach where your partner can go for a swim. If your partner feels the need to stop and identify every bird in the treetops, you can take those moments to check the map, have a drink, or take a few pictures.

Standing around getting bored and angry won't help anything, so go out of your way to enjoy yourself. If your partner has indulged one of your hobbies, be sure to say thanks—either with words or, better yet, with actions.

Making sure you both get to do what you love involves planning. Don't set tight timelines if you need photography or bird-watching breaks 10 times a day. If you need to go for a swim every day to be happy, make sure your campsites will all be on the water's edge. Making all of the "extra" activities part of your plan also lets your partner know what to expect. If he or she knows from the start that you want to spend half a day rock climbing in a specific spot, then you won't be arguing about it when you get there. Your partner can plan for it ahead of time by either joining the climb, or having something else to do, like reading a book or going for a hike.

Share Your Dreams—and Your Concerns

Obviously, communication is the key to planning a trip that will make both of you happy. One of the great things about camping together is the chance to share your dreams. If you've always wanted to see the aurora borealis, or stand on top of Mt. Rainier, then it becomes all the more special to do it with the one person in the world who means the most to you. Talk about the things you'd like to see and do, and find out which ones you both share. If you have a lot of dreams in common, make a list and every time you take a camping vacation together, you can cross something off.

If you're just getting to know someone, communication is even more important. You may be excited about your new partner who loves going on canoe trips as much as you do. But on your first trip together, you may discover that the serene weekend on a lake you had in mind is not a match with the whitewater adventure she had in mind. Clearly, more discussion was needed before the trip.

By deciding ahead of time what you each hope to get out of the trip, you're much more likely to actually accomplish those things. Surprises are fun, but they can also lead to disappointment if your partner doesn't react the way you had hoped.

The dreams you share can take on many forms. They can include places you'd like to see, activities you'd like to learn, or even new additions to your love life. If you're bringing camping into your relationship in hopes of spicing up your sex life, that's something your partner should understand before you head out. If you have outdoor sexual fantasies, for instance, it's a great idea to share those ahead of time so your partner will understand what you have in mind. You can even bring along helpful props or costumes. Have you always wanted to play Adam and Eve? You won't need much for that one, except maybe an apple. What about "seduced by a mermaid" or "captured by a pirate"? All you really need is an isolated spot and your imagination. But if it would help to bring along an eye patch, well, why not!

Sharing your dreams and goals is a great step toward making your trip memorable, but it's also important to share any concerns you may have before you go. If you think the route you are looking at is beyond your skills, speak up before you get too far into your preparations. It might be your partner's dream to kayak down the Colorado River, but if you aren't ready to handle the rapids, then maybe that dream will have to be put on hold until you have enough experience. It's tempting to agree to what your partner wants, just to make him or her happy. But if you are in the middle of the trip unable to continue, or angry with your partner for putting you in this uncomfortable situation, then you'll have nobody to blame but yourself.

How to Even Things Out

We all like to think that we've got a good balance in our relationships. But for a lot of couples, there is an imbalance of some kind that comes into play when you're outdoors together, and it has nothing to do with a bad relationship. Maybe one of you has been camping forever, and the other is a beginner. Or one is significantly taller than the other, or stronger or more fit. All of these things can get in the way of enjoying the same trip, but there are ways to help even things out.

The previous chapter covered a number of ways to help out a beginner. Generally, it's up to the more experienced person to make sure the less experienced person will be comfortable with what's going on. But there are some ways to help push things forward a bit. If you have a lot of trust between you, the less experienced person may be OK with letting the more experienced one navigate a difficult route. Or on a canoe trip, the more experienced person can offer to do all of the steering, so all the beginner has to do is paddle. If you go out together often enough, the beginner's skills will eventually catch up, and you can go on more challenging trips. It takes a bit of patience, but just keep telling yourselves that nobody stays a beginner forever.

That's all fine, but if your partner is a foot taller than you, there's not much chance you're ever going to catch up. (Although, between you and me, I'm still hoping for a midlife growth spurt.) I know it's not politically correct to say so, but size matters, particularly on hikes or backpacking trips. Taller people have a longer stride, so they generally go faster than short people. They also have an easier time climbing up or down slopes, because they can simply step over things that a smaller person has to climb or scramble over. This often leaves the smaller partner working harder, getting more tired, and struggling to keep up. Or it means the taller partner is constantly waiting.

Rock climbing also depends a lot on your build. Having a longer reach can be a huge advantage when holds are scarce. People with a heavier build find climbing much more tiring than their leaner counterparts. And your differences will be hard to ignore if you're roped together.

There are some ways to get on more of an even pace with your partner, even if a growth spurt never materializes.

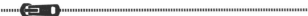

The Grumpy *Mountaineer*

66 When I met Jay, I was really excited because he was a mountaineer. I wanted to do more outdoor stuff, and I thought, "Now I've met a guy who's into that, who will teach me." But when we went out hiking together, he acted bored and miserable. He felt like he was wasting time doing easy stuff with me, when he could be up a mountain somewhere instead, if only I wasn't so inexperienced. He was so hard to be around that I broke up with him after a few months.

Then I met Mike, who was outdoorsy but not so hard-core. He didn't seem to mind "wasting" a weekend hiking with me and giving me advice. Even though he could do much harder stuff, he thought it was OK to take a break from it sometimes. I'll probably never be a mountaineer, but I'm much more confident outdoors than I used to be—but Jay will never know that. **99**

—RW

For backpacking, the taller partner is also usually heavier. When you pack, most people assume that it's fair to divide the weight of your gear evenly between your two packs. In fact, this isn't fair at all. The weight should be divided in proportion to your body weights. Most people who backpack can carry about 25 percent of their weight in a properly fitted pack without too much difficulty. Try to use that as a guideline for how much each of your packs should weigh. For instance, a 200-pound man should be able to carry a 50-pound pack, while his 120-pound partner shouldn't have to take on more than 30 pounds. If you can't pack that light, you'll have to work out who is in better shape and let that person take on the extra punishment.

If weighting your packs by this method still leaves the smaller person trailing behind, then make the difference even greater. Carrying around extra weight will automatically slow you down, and taking weight away will speed you up. Eventually, you will find the balance between the two of you and get yourselves moving at the same pace. Remember that the weight each of you is carrying will change over the course of a multiday trip as you use up some of your food and fuel supplies. So if you are carrying a lot of the food, you might have to add other gear to your pack to keep things fair as the trip goes on.

It can be tough for us women to admit that we can't carry as much weight as our partners, but for our own safety most of us eventually swallow our pride. Like me, Justine has had to face the harsh facts. "I'm 5'2", he's 5'9", so he carries more," she says. "I'm always staunch about us being equal, but when you're two hours into a five-hour slog up a hill—sexual politics don't exist!"

Terrain makes a big difference as well. I'm a lot shorter than Gerhard, but when we're on flat ground, I can keep up with his pace if our packs are weighted correctly. But as soon as the ground is more challenging, it all goes out the window. It takes a lot more effort for me to climb up, down, or over things.

Once, when we were on a four-day trip around a volcanic area of New Zealand, we faced a long climb up a mountain trail that was littered with boulders. Gerhard was ahead of me, and about halfway up, he stopped for a break and let me catch up because some other hikers had gotten between us. "You go up first," he suggested (probably so he could take a longer rest!). As he followed me, he noticed that for every step he took, I had to take two or three to climb over the rocks. Sometimes, I had to use my arms to pull myself up on top of the next boulder.

When we got to the top, he acknowledged that I have to work harder because of my size. "You're at a real disadvantage," he admitted. Now that he has seen me struggle on rough terrain, he respects the extra effort I make whenever I tackle those trails with him.

Paddling a canoe or kayak may seem to be unrelated to size, but that's not entirely true. People with longer arms have a longer, more powerful stroke, particularly in a canoe. If you're trying to match your stroke timing, which can be helpful in a tandem kayak, the person with shorter arms will have to resist the temptation to paddle faster because their strokes are shorter. Sometimes it helps to give the shorter person a slightly longer paddle to compensate. If you each decide to paddle your own boat, you can decide for yourselves how important it is to go the same speed.

Size also matters when selecting a kayak paddle. Women tend to have smaller hands than men, and over a long period of time, it can be very uncomfortable to kayak with a poor-fitting paddle. A paddle with a narrower shaft helps to make things more comfortable for women, or even men with small hands.

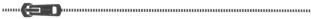

Round and Round We Go

66 My husband and I rented a canoe while we were staying at this beautiful resort in Northern Ontario. Neither of us had used a canoe in years, so we were really wobbly, and I thought for sure we'd end up tipping over. But the most frustrating part was that he has so much more arm strength than me, that with each of us paddling on one side of the canoe, we kept turning toward my side!

I'm sure there's an easy way to make it go straighter, but, like I said, we hadn't done this in years. So he had to keep switching sides while he paddled so we could go in something close to a straight line. I kept trying to match his power, and the next day my arms and shoulders were just killing me. There has to be a better way! **99**

—OB

You should also take your weight into consideration when you pack a canoe or tandem kayak. If one person is lighter, that person should have less of the heavy gear at his or her end of the boat. Use your gear to balance out the load from front to back so the canoe or kayak is as level as possible in the water. This will help to stabilize the boat, particularly if you hit rough water or high winds.

Working as a Team

One of the great things about being in a couple is knowing that someone's got your back. Nobody is just going to stand around while the one they love is getting swept away by a river or is slipping off a cliff. There are many occasions during hiking, camping, paddling, or engaging in other outdoor activities when couples must act as a team, whether they're fording a river or climbing up difficult slopes. By working together, you can keep each other safe and keep an eye on each other at the same time. In fact, building your teamwork skills can be one of the most rewarding parts of camping with your partner. Everything you learn about working as a team out in the wilderness can make you work better together in your everyday life.

Working as a team begins with understanding each other's strengths and weaknesses. Dimitri, a camper from New Zealand, is great when it comes to the technical challenges of backpacking. If he and his girlfriend encounter a tricky route section, he takes charge. "She thinks all trees look alike, and we'll go back along a trail just a few months later, and she won't remember the way at all," he says. "So when there's a question of which way to go, she just defers to me, even if she thinks I've got it wrong." Dimitri also makes a point of showing his girlfriend where they are on the map so that she feels comfortable with the route.

Dimitri may be great at the technical skills, but he's hopeless at logistics. So when it comes to planning and preparation, his girlfriend is chief. She gets all of the gear together, buys the food, and then packs everything neatly and efficiently. "If it was left up to me, I'd be scrambling around at the last minute, trying to cram stuff into packs," Dimitri says. "I even forgot the map once. So now she just makes her lists and checks them twice, and I do whatever she tells me until we leave the house."

It took them a while, but Dimitri and his girlfriend finally developed a system that allows each of them to employ their talents. "We have learned how each other interacts and reacts, and our individual strengths and weaknesses, so we know each other better," he says. "And we encourage each other in the areas we need to strengthen."

They've learned to accept their skills differences and work together. But it can be difficult for many of us to admit we're not so good at something. If your partner is a hopeless navigator or a terrible camp cook, try not to be too judgmental. Hurt feelings can ruin a trip, and aren't really necessary. At the same time, it's important for both of you to be open to honest criticism from your partner. Being defensive about getting lost isn't going to help anything, so if you've made a mistake it's best to admit that you're not perfect.

Janet feels more comfortable camping with her partner because he is very supportive, even when she's trying something new. "He's absolutely non-macho," she says. "He encourages me to do physical things that make me slightly nervous, but he gives me advice on how to tackle the obstacle, and he offers a helping hand if I need it. My former husband nearly put me off backpacking by telling me I wasn't good at it. He put other people down, and I didn't know then that it was a sign of his own insecurities."

One couple I spoke to have a great time camping together, except when it comes time to pitch the tent. "We're usually tired from a long drive out to the campground," says Renee, "and we just want to get the damn thing up so we can start enjoying ourselves. But somehow we just get in each other's way the entire time and make a mess of the whole thing!"

Eventually, they decided that he would put up the tent by himself, and she would take that time to do other tasks, like sorting out the cooking gear and organizing things for the next day. By dividing their tasks, they don't have anything to argue about. "We don't even discuss it anymore," Renee says. "We both just know what needs to be done, and we go ahead and do it. Then by the time the work is all done, we're really happy to spend some time together."

You'll see what you can do best when you work together, and what's easier for one of you to take care of alone. Some couples like to do everything together. It strengthens their bond and makes each chore go a bit faster. This is a good method if one of you is a beginner and is unsure of how to accomplish tasks on your own. It gives the more experienced camper an opportunity to share knowledge, and the beginner an opportunity to be helpful.

Others couples prefer to "divide and conquer" by divvying up the chores and having each person take care of certain things. This works better for a lot of campers who are both experienced but have different ways of doing the same thing. There's no point in arguing about the

Who Says *Chivalry Is Dead?*

66 We have this little thing when there's a river to cross—sacrifice the David. As I am tall and my girlfriend is short, sometimes the rivers are waist deep or higher on her. So I go first and put my pack on the other side, then I take my girlfriend's pack and help her across. By which time, having had my legs immersed in water up to my groin, I can't feel just below the waist. 99

—DM

"right" way to hang the food, as long as the task is accomplished in the end. If you are both competent campers, the divide-and-conquer method is often the fastest way to get everything done.

Some tasks are easier when tackled as a team. When you're faced with a fast-flowing river to cross, for example, it can be easier to keep your footing if the two of you link arms. Working together makes it easier to climb aboard a capsized canoe or kayak, too. One of you can keep the boat balanced while the other climbs in. It takes practice to be an effective team, but the more you get outdoors together, the more your skills will develop as you try different techniques together. Eventually, you may get to the point where you don't even need to discuss what each of you should be doing—you'll just know.

The Blame Game

It's the end of a long day on the water, and you've just set up camp. You light the gas stove to make your much-anticipated dinner. After a few minutes, the stove goes out. You've run out of gas. You ask your partner to get out another fuel bottle. Your partner didn't pack a second fuel bottle, since you didn't tell him the first one was running low. You get mad about your partner's lack of planning. Your partner gets angry about your lack of initiative. Either way, there's no dinner.

Couples rarely fight when things are going well. So as long as your trip is going to plan, you are probably going to have a lovely time together. But as soon as things start to go wrong, the tension can lead to arguments between even the most devoted of couples.

What's the first thing most of us do when something goes wrong? Try to figure out who's to blame. We want to know why we have found ourselves in this bad situation. We want the person who made the mistake to take full responsibility. We want answers, and we want them now! In a camping environment, the cause of the problem is not usually the most important thing to be thinking about.

The first thing to consider is how to fix the situation. You can go back and analyze where things went wrong later. Don't make any rash decisions based on anger or stubbornness. It's not just petty and immature, it's also dangerous.

Try to remember what it is you're arguing about, and stay on topic. Don't call your entire relationship into question just because your partner took a wrong turn at the last fork in the river. It really has nothing to do with how often he plays poker with his college buddies, even if that seems relevant to you at the time. Avoid using phrases that will escalate the discussion into a huge debate. Sweeping accusations like "you always..." or "you never..." are bound to get your partner on the defensive and complicate whatever problems you are facing. Getting off topic or expanding the argument into a broader area means that it will take longer for you to actually resolve the problem at hand (such as being lost) and could even make things worse (such as being lost after dark).

Once you have determined that something is wrong (you are lost, you are missing a piece of gear, one of you is hurt, etc.), stop where you are if it is safe to do so. From there, relax and discuss the situation to make sure that you both understand it the same way. Many couples have an inherent power struggle in their relationship to begin with. This can make it hard for either partner to admit they may be wrong. The standoff is counterproductive, particularly in the wilderness. It's important to come up with a solution you can both accept. Once you agree on a plan of action, you can get up and start solving your problem—together. Don't storm off to find the trail or a lost piece of gear, leaving your partner behind because you don't agree on which way to go. There is safety in numbers, and when there are only two of you, you can't afford to have two different plans to deal with an emergency.

Camping trips are not good times to keep your problems to yourself. If you think you are lost, it's important to tell your partner right away, rather than getting anxious

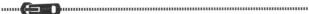

And Another Thing . . .

66 When my girlfriend, Emma, and I decided to take up hiking, I thought it would be relaxing and give us a break from all the bickering we do normally. It took exactly half a day to prove that theory wrong! I had a trail map, and I was trying to follow it, but there were a lot of branches, and at some point we hit a dead-end.

Emma started in on me right away: "This is so typical of you. You just had to be the one with the map, didn't you?!" I didn't see how this could be "typical" of me since it was our first hike, and I told her so. She then started yelling at me for always having to be in charge all the time, and not ever listening to anything she ever had to say.

By this point, I was getting pissed off, and I started to ask her a string of those rhetorical questions that are inadvisable in relationship spats. "Did you say we were going the wrong way? No! Did you offer to take the map? No! You never want to be in charge because you never want to be the responsible one!"

We must have fought there for at least 20 minutes until eventually we saw another group of hikers. I asked them to point out where we were on the map, and we found our way back to the car from there.

I don't know how long we would have stood there fighting about our relationship if those other people didn't come along. My God, we'd probably still be there! 99

—NP

about it for an hour while your partner diligently follows you. If you don't feel well, share this information, too. It will certainly help your partner to know that you were a bit dizzy and nauseous all day, if you suddenly pass out

and can't say a word. If you talk about problems as they come up, there is a good chance you can work them out before they become arguments or emergencies. (That said, true emergencies are not good times to delve into relationship issues, as we'll discuss next.)

Leave Your Problems at Home

Almost every couple has something going on that's bugging them. Going on a camping trip together can be a great way to escape from your daily routine and the problems you're facing together. It gives you something else to focus on, and takes you out of the situations that may normally start arguments, like looking at the pile of bills on the table. This is why so many couples feel that camping together revitalizes their relationships and keeps the romance alive.

It's far too easy to spoil this escape by dragging the problems of your home life out into the wilderness with you. Think of the camping trip as a clean break from everything at home. Make an agreement to stay away from certain topics before you leave. There's nothing you can do about paying off your credit card or fixing your leaky roof while you're out camping, so there's no point in bringing it up. Make a conscious decision to live in the moment and enjoy a bit of time away from all of those worries. If you should find yourselves starting to bicker, stop and have a look around. Where are you? What are you missing by not even taking in your surroundings? The most romantic settings can be taken for granted if you're too absorbed in your problems to enjoy them. You made the effort to get outdoors into a place of natural beauty—don't waste it!

If you know that certain topics always cause arguments, try to ban them from your camping trips. This is a method that a lot of people use when they are trying to lose weight. There are certain "trigger" foods they know they have trouble controlling their portions with, and those foods are banned. Whatever you know will lead to

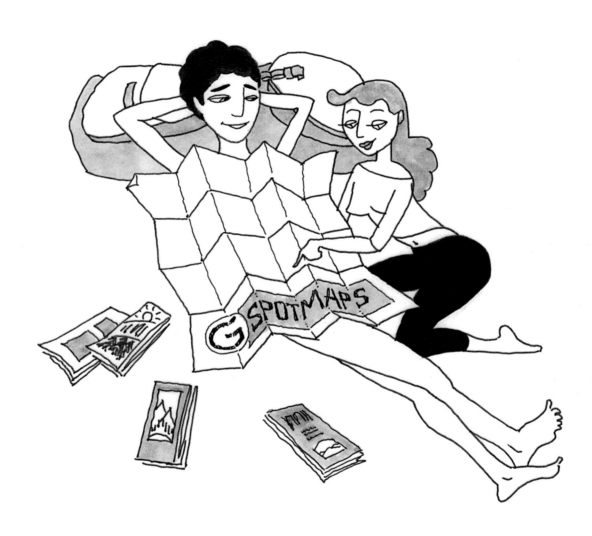

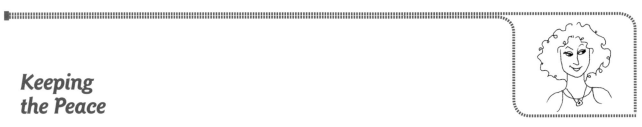

Keeping the Peace

If you and your partner always seem to be getting into arguments on your trips, here are some tips for making things go a bit smoother.

GET INTO A ROUTINE. Once you've found a way to pitch the tent, or set up the campsite, or make breakfast, that works for the two of you, do it the same way every trip. If you have a routine, you'll always meet each other's expectations and there will be nothing to fight about.

SYMPATHIZE. When your partner slips and falls crossing a river, then emerges covered in green slime, you might feel compelled to have a good laugh over it. Instead, ask your partner if he or she is hurt, and express your sympathy if you partner is feeling sore or frightened by the experience. This goes for any situation when something unplanned happens to your partner. Let the victim decide whether it's funny, and then follow suit. If your partner isn't laughing, you shouldn't be, either.

DO IT WITHOUT BEING ASKED. Nobody likes to be nagged, so don't give your partner a reason to do it. If you see that something needs to be done (like fetching more water or washing the dishes), just take the initiative and do it. Instead of getting nagged, you'll find you're getting thanked!

IF YOU DON'T HAVE ANYTHING NICE TO SAY, DON'T SAY ANYTHING. You probably learned this when you were 5, but it's the kind of advice that sometimes gets forgotten under stress. Unless it is a matter of safety, don't criticize your partner for doing something differently from how you do it. Encouragement is a lot more helpful than criticism.

IF YOU DON'T HAVE ANYTHING TO SAY, SAY SOMETHING NICE. Yes, the opposite actually works, too! When everything is going OK and is under control, there might not seem to be a need to talk about it. But as I said, encouragement is helpful. When things are calm, give your partner an unsolicited compliment. I guarantee you'll get a smile, and it will put you both in a good mood.

BE PREPARED. Those Boy Scouts got it right. Try to foresee the challenges you may be facing on your trip, and go with a plan already in place to deal with them. That way, you won't have the added stress of coming up with a plan in the middle of the wild.

GIVE EACH OTHER SPACE. Some couples don't do well with being together 24/7. If that sounds like you, find ways to spend some time apart during your camping trips. When it's not essential to stick together (like when you're in the same canoe, or following a tricky trail), you can do other activities on your own—reading, swimming, sketching, or whatever puts you in a good head space.

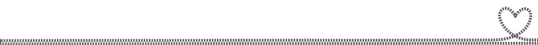
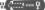

a long, painful argument should be off limits. Stay away from your trigger issues. They'll be right where you left them when you get home, but at least you'll be refreshed and hopefully better prepared to deal with them.

Camping together should bring you closer as a couple, not drive you apart. But it takes planning and effort, just like the rest of your relationship. And as always, the key to success is good communication. The more you share, the more likely you are to plan a trip that you will both enjoy and cherish together. Even the problems you face can serve to strengthen your relationship, as long as you remember to work as a team and forget about the blame. Learning to trust and rely on one another is one of the most special achievements a couple can bring to their relationship through camping.

A final thought: The end of a tiring day is the most common time for couples to start bickering. So give some thought to your arrival time at camp when you plan a trip. Getting to your campsite after sundown and trying to set up the tent and make dinner in the dark can lead to a lot of frustration. If you can, plan to arrive in daylight so you can get yourselves comfortable and organized. If you know that won't be possible, pack your equipment so that your tent, flashlights, food, and cooking gear are exactly where you expect them to be. Don't make yourselves go digging through everything in the dark. You're bound to have trouble finding something and get into a fight about who put it away in the wrong place.

Chapter 3:

How to Keep Smelling

GOOD ENOUGH TO KISS

Often when a bunch of guys go on a camping trip together, they think that part of the fun is wearing the same smelly socks for the whole trip and farting in the tent. Groups of girls aren't much better, except that they're less likely to try to put out the embers of their campfire by peeing on them. (Ouch!)

When Gerhard and I went on our first camping trip together, it was early in our relationship. I was at that stage in the relationship when I felt like I had to look my best when we went out together. I was still trying to make a good impression. But camping was going to make that impossible. He would see me getting all sweaty, with no makeup. He would see my hair unwashed and unstyled. I'd be wearing my unflattering hiking pants with the zip-off legs. After obsessing about it for longer than I care to admit, I finally decided that if he still wants to sleep with me after all of that, there's hope for the future of this relationship.

A camping trip is by no means the time for mascara, cologne, or hair gel, but a bit of grooming can make a huge difference in your sex appeal after a few days in the wilderness. If you're going to be with your partner, you've got to take into account how you look—*and* how you smell.

Your hair is not going to look great after the first day away from a mirror, so don't even bother trying. You'll probably need a hat to protect you from the sun or rain anyway, and they're great for covering up messy hair. Most long-haired campers use ponytails or braids to keep their hair tidy and out of the way. Using hair spray or other products to keep things in order is only going to attract bugs, so give up on your perfect hair for a few days and stick with the hat and the ponytail.

I've run into groups of teenagers on camping trips, and there are always a few of them trying to keep looking "cute" while they're out in the wilderness. They religiously apply lip gloss, and they wear hair clips with little rhinestones all over them. I've even caught some of the boys trying to fix their hair in whatever reflective surface they could find. I get it; looking good is important when you're trying to impress your peers. And it's not just the kids who do it. Kiwi camper Justine admitted to me that she can't let go of her girlie side when she hits the trails. "Just because you're tramping doesn't mean you can't look glamorous," she says. "I always wear a flower clip in my hair. My partner laughs every time I make a beauty stop to rearrange my hair. Sometimes I take a photo of myself with our digital camera just so I can play it back."

Val, on the other hand, finds that a little pre-trip preparation can make her feel sexier while she's away from civilization. "Before I leave on a trip, I have my hair done, my legs and bikini line waxed, and feet pedicured and varnished in a pretty, funky color," she says. "I even get my eyelashes tinted. No, really! It makes a vast difference to my self-confidence." Is she just a misplaced city girl? Nope, she's been camping for decades. "I am honestly a very experienced and enthusiastic hiker, but you will not find me leaving without these preparations," she says.

I'm even guilty of wilderness vanity myself. I'm far more likely to buy a new hiking shirt if I think it looks cute on me. I'll go for the v-neck instead of the crew neck because it shows off my cleavage. And I'm pretty sure I'm not the only one, because I've noticed that outdoor clothing is getting more and more attractive. Items like thong underwear have started appearing in camping shops, along with form-fitting, color-coordinated outfits for every type of activity. Fashion invaded surfing culture way back in the '60s, and now it's caught up with us campers.

Dressing for Success

What you wear can make a huge difference not only in terms of how you look, but, perhaps more importantly, in how you smell. There comes a point in every trip when I catch a nasty scent in the air and realize in horror that it's me! That's my cue to find somewhere to get cleaned up before I try for any kind of intimacy that night.

Choosing the right fabrics and layers is the key to smelling better (or at least less horrible) for longer. Synthetic

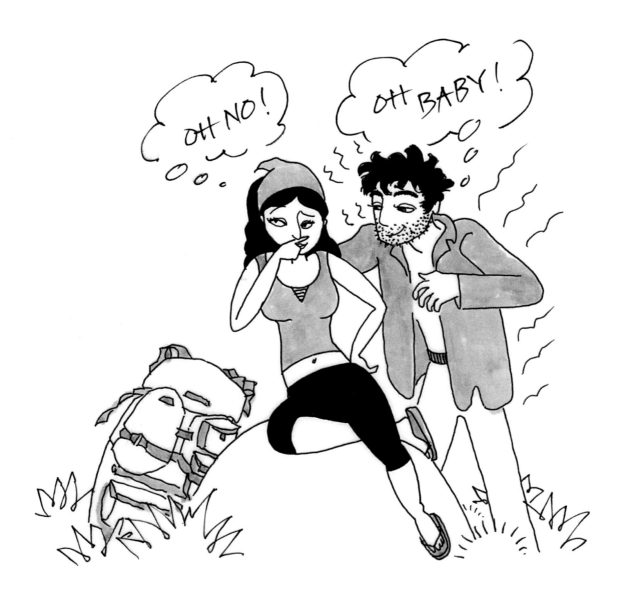

fabrics like polypropylene and polyester are good for wicking away the sweat from your body, so most campers like to wear them. But after a day or two, they start to smell pretty strong—sort of like sour milk mixed with a hint of wet fur. While it doesn't make sense to sacrifice warmth or comfort just so you can smell nice, if you're heading on a longer trip, bring along two shirts that serve as a first layer and wash one of them with a bit of biodegradable soap every couple of days. Even without water, giving one of your shirts the chance to air out for a day can make it smell much better. Cotton T-shirts are not a good idea for anyone who sweats a lot (or for outdoor-wear in general). They absorb the sweat, making the clothing not only wet and uncomfortable but also stinky.

A lot of campers claim that wool tops are the best for resisting the stink, and wool can be worn for three or four sweaty days before it gets smelly. Some people find wool irritating next to their skin, but fine, soft knits are now widely available and shouldn't feel like your old, scratchy sweater. Merino wool, in particular, has caught on as both a base layer and a middle layer.

Even if your clothing does get a bit ripe after the first few days, you can make things more pleasant for you and your partner by changing your clothes when you make camp for the night. As soon as you're done with the sweaty work for the day, put on some dry, clean clothes. Have one shirt, one pair of socks and, if possible, one pair of pants or long johns that you wear only at the campsites. That way, they will never get sweaty or wet, and you'll always be nice and huggable when it comes time to bed down.

Sweat isn't the only issue when you choose your camping clothes. After all, into all our lives, a little rain must fall! Choosing the right stuff for wet weather will keep you from being completely miserable, and because weatherproof clothes will keep you dry, they'll also keep you from smelling like a wet dog.

Monique's husband learned that lesson the hard way. "When we started camping, my husband didn't see the point in buying a lot of expensive new clothing made especially for the outdoors," she says. "He figured it was all a big rip-off and he'd be perfectly fine in his regular clothes."

He changed his tune the first time they got hit with a downpour during a camping weekend. "He was wearing jeans, an old sweatshirt, and an old, rubbery rain jacket that didn't breathe," she says. "His jeans were soaked, and they didn't dry out for the rest of the trip, so he was constantly cold. The rain jacket made him sweat so much that his sweatshirt also got soaked." By the time they planned their next trip, he had invested in some quick-dry nylon pants and a fleece pullover. Eventually, he even forked out the big bucks for a Gore-Tex jacket.

Of course, when you're on a romantic camping trip with your partner, you want to look good as well as smell good. And although warmth and comfort are the most important qualities to consider when choosing your camping clothes, you don't have to sacrifice sexiness in the process. In recent years, some companies have begun to take appearance into consideration, too. According to the folks who make and sell outdoor clothes, it's women who have brought style to the wilderness.

"The awful truth is that for many years, women's sizes of outdoor clothing were often really more like unisex sizes, with predictable effects on fit and function," says Philip Torrens, who works for the Canadian outdoor retailer Mountain Equipment Co-op. "Manufacturers finally wised up to the fact that they were ill-serving at least half their potential market and began making clothing truly sized for women. And behold: Not only does the new clothing make the women look less like workers from a Soviet-era farm collective, it also improves performance. Clothing that actually fits well doesn't trip, bind, or otherwise impede hiking and climbing." (Another plus is that it attracts sexual attention!)

Beaver Theodosakis, founder of Prana, the Prada of outdoor clothing, adds, "For most people, women's lines were an afterthought. For us, (the women's clothing

Nice Ways to Say, "You Stink!"

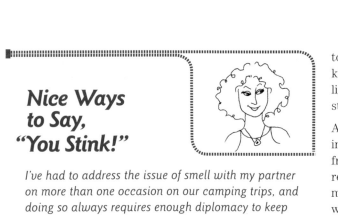

I've had to address the issue of smell with my partner on more than one occasion on our camping trips, and doing so always requires enough diplomacy to keep from offending him, with enough force to get him to clean up his act. Having trouble with your approach?

Try out some of these lines:

Wow, honey, you're really starting to get that "woodsy" smell.

You worked pretty hard today, and these moist wipes are really refreshing.

This looks like a nice place for a swim. Why don't you join me?

I bet if we rinse that shirt out, it will dry completely by the fire tonight.

Would you like to borrow my toothpaste?

How about we switch places? I prefer to be upwind.

Maybe you should change your clothes before you go to sleep.

Do you smell something funny in here?

I'm sure your feet will feel better if you cool them off in the water.

Take off your clothes so I can wet you down, baby!

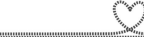

range) has gone from 25 percent (of our sales) to about 65 percent. The girls, if they like something, they'll buy one in every color." Prana offers fashion-friendly choices to their female customers by making their clothes in all kinds of fun colors and patterns, instead of the traditional light and dark khaki range that used to be the camping standard.

And it's not just the women who are pushing the change in outdoor fashion. Prana got a call several years ago from male rock climber Chris Sharma. Although he already had a clothing sponsor, he was attracted to Prana's more fashionable look. "He called us to say, 'I want to wear your clothing. Whenever I'm in my climbing stuff, I feel like I'm on the set of a Star Trek movie!'" Theodosakis recalls. Theodosakis and the design team at Prana were more than happy to make sure that Sharma looks like a hunky earthling at all times.

All of this fashion influence doesn't mean that you shouldn't dress for the activity and the weather. "People could have a turtleneck, hat, and gloves on and be sexy," Theodosakis says. "It's an attitude."

It's not just Prana who has picked up on the demand for sexy outdoor attire. Outdoor clothing companies like Patagonia, Columbia, North Face, and Helly Hansen are all offering more fashionable ranges of clothing than ever before. Brands from retail chains like REI and MEC are also in on the movement. It has come to the point where you could actually arrive back in the city after a camping trip and not look out of place hitting the town.

So be picky about your camping clothes. Get the right technical fabrics to keep you warm (or cool), comfortable, and dry. Choose items that will keep you from getting too stinky, or that are easy to wash and dry. And on top of all that, you should be able to find something that looks good on you, so you'll feel sexy no matter how long you've been away from your city wardrobe.

No More Stinky Feet

Anyone who has a partner with stinky feet knows that you don't want to be stuck in a tent with those feet overnight. If they stink under normal conditions, just imagine how bad they'll smell after hiking all day, or wearing the same socks for a few days. And what if they're also covered in blisters and growing fungus? There's nothing sexy about that! Beyond smell, foot care is important for everyone; blisters or athlete's foot can really ruin a camping trip if they get out of hand (or, in this case, foot).

Some hikers swear by the layered-sock method to prevent blisters. Start with a thin liner sock, which will wick away the sweat, and top that with a thicker sock to prevent boots or shoes from rubbing. The double-sock approach works well for people whose feet sweat a lot. Not only will it help prevent blisters, but if you bring two pairs of liner socks, you can rinse one of them out each day to keep the stink under control without having to pack a second pair of thicker hiking socks. Personally, I'm happy to wear one pair of good, wicking socks. I like to keep things as simple as possible.

If you've been in sweaty hiking socks all day, change out of them and put on clean, dry socks as soon as you arrive at camp. This will give your hiking socks a chance to dry or air out. (Hang them outside so they don't stink up the tent.) It's a good idea to rinse or wash your feet when you change socks. It will keep your camp socks cleaner, and your feet won't smell when you go to bed. If you keep putting on your same dirty, stinky socks during the day, you'll always have your clean, dry pair to use at night. People who try to rotate between two pairs of socks on alternating days usually just end up with two pairs of wet, dirty socks and no clean, dry ones. Of course, some people like to bring a fresh pair of socks for every day, but the longer your trip, the more ridiculous that gets. If you're going to be camping for a week, let's assume you have more important things to fit into your pack than seven pairs of thick hiking socks.

There's not much point in changing into nice, clean socks at the campsite if you shove them back into your wet, smelly hiking boots. It's better to have another pair of shoes to wear around camp so you can give your feet a break, and give your hiking boots (or water shoes) a chance to dry and air out overnight. Sandals are great camp shoes because they are small and light to pack, and they let your feet breathe so they won't start to sweat again. Lightweight plastic clogs like Crocs are popular with campers these days. They're nice and comfy and don't weigh a thing, plus they can get wet and you just wipe them dry.

If you're on a paddling trip, odds are that you'll be spending your days in sandals, water slippers, or bare feet. You have a big advantage over the hikers when it comes to keeping your feet clean since you can just stick them in the water whenever you want. On the other hand, because your footwear is wet a lot of the time, you'll have to wash your shoes with soap now and then to stop mold from growing. Take them off to do this, so you can scrub any gunk off of the footbeds. It's amazing how bad sandals can smell if they never get cleaned (one friend refers to this as "Teva funk").

If your partner is too lax about clean feet, and you can't take the stench, try a bit of motivation. If freshly washed feet are rewarded with a foot rub, it might just seem worth the bother after all.

How to Wash Without a Shower in Sight

Some car camping areas have actual shower facilities, but for backpackers, paddlers, and other backcountry travelers, a bit of rustic ingenuity is needed. Keeping yourself clean on a camping trip is often a case of using whatever opportunities present themselves, but forward thinking helps, too. Not only will washing now and then keep you smelling better, it's also a great opportunity to spend some time naked with your partner!

Most campsites are close to a source of water, either a river or a lake. If there is fresh water nearby, and the weather is good, the easiest way to wash is to go for a swim. It will feel great after a long day of paddling or hiking, and it will give you a chance to have some together time. If you're reasonably secluded, skinny-dipping is

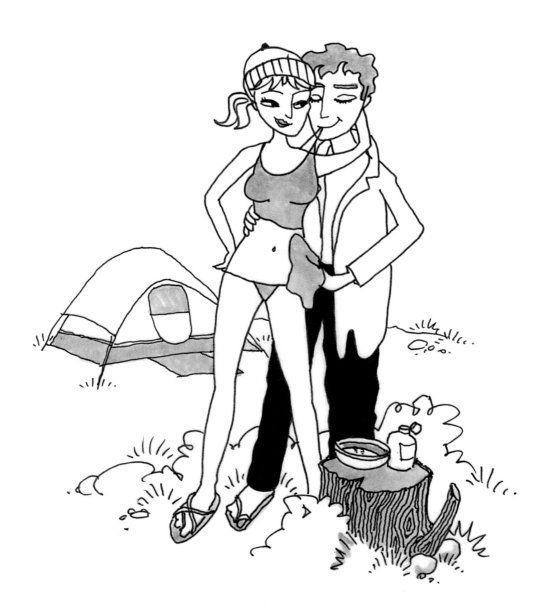

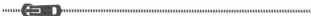

Acting Dirty,
Getting Clean

66 I don't think that staying clean when we're camping is a problem. We do most of our camping in Algonquin Park in Northern Ontario, which is just full of water. Actually, washing can be the highlight of our day. After a long hike, we'll usually make a point of getting a campsite near a lake.

If we're alone, we'll go in and bathe naked, but if it's a more popular lake and there are people around, we'll wear bathing suits. We bring a washcloth with us, and then one of us will wash the other and give them a massage at the same time. Then we trade places. We get nice and clean and soothe our aching muscles at the same time.

Then sometimes if we know there's nobody around, we'll have sex up on the shore on one of our towels, and then run back into the water afterward to rinse off. I always feel like we're getting away with something bad, but in a good way—if that makes sense. **99**

—MR

great fun. I think it's most romantic to go skinny-dipping after dark, by moonlight. It also makes me less nervous about someone else coming by and seeing me naked. One of the most amazing experiences I've ever had was a late-night swim under the aurora borealis, or northern lights. It was so magical floating under a sky that was alive with color. Moments like that are unforgettable, and they don't cost a cent.

Bathing in a lake or river is lovely, but don't forget the cardinal rule of camping—take nothing but pictures and leave nothing but footprints. Chemical residue from soaps and shampoos can be very harmful to the natural environment. If you want to soap up, use only biodegrad-

able soaps and shampoos, available in most camping stores. Even the biodegradable soap shouldn't go straight into the water source, but should be used on shore and rinsed away at least 200 feet from the water source.

If the water near your campsite is too cold for a swim, or not deep enough, you can clean up using a camp shower. Camp showers are a fabulous invention. They consist of a large, plastic bladder, which is usually black, and a rubber hose with a small, water-diffusing spout. You just fill up the bladder with water, and leave it in the sun for an hour or more. The dark plastic attracts and holds heat, making the water warm. (On a sunny day, you can actually end up with a hot shower!) Hang the bladder from a tree branch and open the valve for the spout. These take up a bit of extra space, but they are quite light and a great little luxury item for a long trip.

Even without an "official" shower, you can improvise using your drinking bladder with its hose. If the weather isn't warm enough to heat up your water, you can warm it on your camp stove first. (Make sure it's not too hot for your bladder before you transfer it in.) Then hang your bladder from a tree and you're good to go.

Since you've got to hang the shower from a tree anyway, it's easy enough to find a wooded area that will shield you from prying eyes so you can throw a little sexy fun into the experience. You can have standing sex against the tree and not even have to move to wash up—it's shower sex with a tree-hugger twist!

If you don't want to hang a shower, use a collapsible bowl or sink instead. They hold quite a bit of water and can be used as a wash basin at your campsite. There are inflatable plastic models, as well as waterproof fabric ones. Of course, any old camping pot will also work. In this scenario, you'll want to enlist your partner's help to scrub your back. A small washcloth or towel is handy.

If your trip is hit with a rainy day, you can turn that to your advantage as well. One couple, Ben and Cristina, told me about a canoe trip they took in which the weather got ugly. "The first day, we were feeling all smug because it was just a bit of rain and everyone else seemed to have decided to stay home," says Ben. "We were cruising down the river, and there was nobody to be seen anywhere. By the time we went to sleep that night, it was starting to rain a little heavier, but we were warm and cozy by then, so we didn't mind."

They woke to pouring rain, with no signs of it stopping any time soon. They weren't more than a couple hours' paddle from their next campsite, so they decided to wait it out in the tent. Eventually, they got stir crazy and decided to embrace the weather instead of hiding from it. "We stripped off our clothes and went outside in just our sandals," says Ben. "There was nobody else around the campsite or on the river. We got our shower stuff and took a shower in the rain. It was actually a lot of fun! If it's going to rain, we figured we might as well put it to good use."

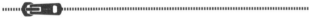

You Kiss Your Mother with that Mouth?

66 I honestly don't think about keeping clean that much while I'm out camping. But every once in a while, my girlfriend will say, "When was the last time you brushed your teeth?" That's her subtle way of telling me that my breath stinks and she's not going anywhere near me until I do something about it. She's even started carrying around those little mouthwash strips in the pocket of her hiking shorts so that when we stop for lunch or a snack we can freshen up afterwards. She says kissing someone with bad breath is like licking the inside of a garbage can. I guess you can't get much more clear than that. Message received! **99**

—GL

They turned what could have been a depressing canoe trip into one of their favorite camping memories just by having a sense of adventure. It never stopped raining that whole weekend, but they had a great time anyway.

If you are camped too far from a water source to use it for cleaning, or you only have saltwater around, you may have to find other ways to clean up. Packing some Wet Ones or baby wipes in a sealed baggie is an easy way to have a quick wash. These are pre-wetted towels that won't force you to use any of your precious drinking water for bathing. They're also handy for winter camping, when getting completely wet may not seem like such a great idea. A quick wipe down of your smelliest parts will make you feel much better, and your partner will be more likely to get close to you. It's also a good idea to use one of them before going to bed, to wipe off the day's sunscreen and bug repellent before you start kissing it off of each other. Not only do those lotions taste bad, they're pretty potent chemicals that you don't want to swallow.

Taking Care of Your Breath

Have you ever leaned in for a nice, romantic smooch and had your partner pull away, or give you the old closed-mouth kiss? Keeping your breath fresh on a camping trip is simple, and it will make a big difference in how many kisses you'll get. Most campers find it easy enough to carry a toothbrush and toothpaste.

Carry a small, travel-sized tube of toothpaste to save bulk and weight. But beware of flip-up caps: These can come open inside your pack and make a huge mess. Screw-on lids are much safer.

During the day, you can give your breath a boost by keeping some mints or gum handy. Try to bring a package of mints with a good closure, so they don't spill all over your pockets or your pack. I've come home from trips and ended up picking fuzzy mints out of my backpack for days. Not into mint? Cinnamon hearts are another breath saver. There's a reason these little guys are so popular on Valentine's Day. The smell of cinnamon is traditionally thought to be an aphrodisiac. So look out, because cinnamon kisses could lead to a lot more!

At night, you can also freshen your breath by drinking a cup of strong peppermint tea. This will leave your whole mouth minty fresh. If you're feeling adventurous, mint tea has other uses. If you have a cup of it with you while performing oral sex, the combination of your heated mouth and the coolness of the menthol have an intense stimulating effect on your partner's sensitive genital skin. It works for both men and women. Just take a mouthful every minute or so and swish it around before you swallow it. If you're going down on a man, you can try to leave a bit of the tea in your mouth (as long as it's not too hot) and let it drip over his penis. Tea time will never be the same!

Girl Stuff

OK, men, you can skip ahead to the next chapter. Girls, there's some stuff you need to know about before you go into the woods. It's the stuff your partner doesn't ever think about because he just doesn't have to deal with it.

Peeing in the Woods

Men have it easy. They can just wander off to the side of the trail and unzip. It's enough to give you penis envy! For girls, having a pee when there's no toilet around can be a logistical nightmare. When I started camping, I had no idea how to handle peeing without a toilet. It was a bit like going through toilet training all over again. Do you have any idea how hard it is to reach into your pocket for toilet paper when you're squatting and dripping, and your pants (and pockets) are around your ankles? I ended up learning some tricks by reading Kathleen Meyer's book *How to Shit in the Woods*, which has a peeing section that helped to clarify things for me. After that, I was able to develop my own preferences, and I always remember to take the paper out of my pocket first. I hope this section will be just as helpful to you. Like any skill, once you know the basics, it gets a lot easier.

You might be tempted to try to hold out for the next available outhouse, but sometimes there just isn't one for hours. Some trails are so remote that there won't be any outhouses on your entire trip. Besides, holding it in can lead to bladder infections, and you don't want one of those while you're camping.

The main goal here is to hit the ground and nothing else (like your feet or your pants) when you pee. The key is gravity. Your pee will fall to the lowest available point, and you want to make sure that's not where your feet are planted. There are a few ways to make this easier.

METHOD 1: ROCKS OR LOGS

If the area has some larger rocks, or medium-sized fallen trees, you can use these to get you off the ground. Find or arrange either two large rocks, or two fallen trees, with a gap at least 4 inches wide between them. Place one foot on each rock or tree (make sure they're stable!), then drop your pants and squat, peeing into the gap. This keeps your feet off the ground and out of the way. There is a seated variation of this method for women who aren't big on balancing. You can put your feet up on one rock or log while your bum rests on another rock.

METHOD 2: GOING WITH THE FLOW

If you are on a slope, your pee will travel downhill. It is easiest to use this method if there is a strong tree nearby, particularly if the hill is steep. Stand on the downhill side of the tree, facing the trunk. Drop your pants and squat, holding onto the tree trunk for support and balance. Make sure your bottom is thrust backward so you don't hit your underpants.

METHOD 3: DIG A HOLE

If there are no hills, logs, or rocks available, it's time to make your own little toilet. Use a small shovel or trowel (which you'll need for burying solid waste if you're camping away from outhouses) to dig a small hole a few inches deep. If you don't have a proper tool, you will have to use a strong stick, or even your hands. Once you have your hole, drop your pants and squat over it, peeing into the hole. Your pee will be trapped in the hole, eventually getting absorbed into the soil, and it won't run all over the ground and your feet.

The only place these methods may fail you is on solid rock or ice. In that case, look for a small crack or crevice to squat over, and do the best you can.

While researching this book, one woman told me she liked to pee by hanging off the edge of a picnic table. I don't know about you, but I would not have dinner with this woman! Keep your "toilet" away from your cooking and eating locations. If there's no outhouse near your campsite, you should pick a spot to use that's at least 100 feet away from where you're going to cook.

METHOD 4: THE FUNNEL

For those women who would prefer to be like men for that crucial moment, some products on the market can help you to pee while standing up. You can get a funnel-shaped device that you hold under your vagina, and it will direct the stream of urine to the ground in front of you. There are disposable versions with different designs, including the Whizzy and the P-Mate. These are made for one use only, so you'd have to bring a bunch of them with you on a camping trip and throw them away when you get back to a trash can. There are plastic versions, like the Shewee or the TravelMate, which can be washed and reused as many times as you like. You can even throw a Shewee in the dishwasher or washing machine when you get home.

The main drawbacks to these devices are keeping them clean so they don't smell, and having to keep them somewhere handy all day. If you are using one of these, bring your water bottle with you whenever you go to pee so you can rinse it out after each use (which means you should also carry extra water), unless you're happy to carry it around in its used state. And be sure to carry it in a sealable plastic bag so it doesn't contaminate anything else.

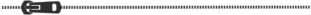

Who Hid the Trees?

66 I've been camping for a long, long time, so I thought I was ready for just about anything. No "girlie" issues for me. But then my first time backpacking in the desert was pretty much a nightmare. I was used to camping in the woods and being able to hide among the trees whenever I needed to pee. But suddenly I was in a place with no trees! I couldn't figure out where to hide.

I held it in for ages, and then finally got desperate enough to duck behind a large rock and hope nobody was coming from that side. After the first day, I realized that the odds of someone else wandering by as I was having a pee were pretty slim, so I would just go behind the scrub or a large rock and have my husband stand guard while I did my thing. I have to admit, though, it made me feel "girlie." 99

—MR

Once you've chosen a technique to try, make sure you're ready to wipe when you're done. As I learned, balancing on rocks is enough of a challenge without simultaneously trying to find your toilet paper. In an ideal world, you should use a handful of grass or soft leaves to wipe yourself after you pee. These are a natural part of the environment and won't do any damage to the ecosystem. This is most important in places with a lot of human traffic, since there could be an awful lot of toilet paper left around otherwise. Of course, you should always check the ground for poison ivy and other irritating plants before you stop to pee, but double-check again before you grab a handful of leaves to wipe with. I can't imagine a worse place for a poison ivy rash!

If that's a little closer to nature than you can handle, go ahead and use tissues or toilet paper. Just don't leave it lying around afterwards. Either pack it out (the preferred method) or bury your used paper in a shallow hole, where it will eventually biodegrade and become part of the soil. Some people try to burn their toilet paper, but it can easily blow away while it's on fire and start a real blaze. Unless you're completely surrounded by rock, sand, or snow, don't take the risk. If you want to burn it, pack it with you and throw it in your campfire at night. You may want to wait until after you've done any cooking over the fire.

These same rules apply if you have to pass solids as well as liquids. You should always dig a hole about 6 inches deep for your solid waste, and bury it along with the leaves or toilet paper when you're done. Remember, other people may step off the trail in the same area, and they won't appreciate coming across your poo!

However you decide to relieve yourself, make sure you choose a spot that is far enough from the trail, and from any water source that campers or animals might use. Popular trails can see thousands upon thousands of campers every year, and it's easy for the trail to get polluted by careless visitors who can't be bothered to take more than a few steps before watering the bushes. Well-used beaches where paddlers stop to eat and rest can suffer even more from a concentration of evacuations. So take those extra steps away from high-use areas.

If you're one of those women who must pee 20 times a day, you might want to work on your bladder-control skills before you go into the woods. Sound silly? It's easier than you might think. By strengthening the pubococcygeal, or PC, muscles on the pelvic floor, you'll have an easier time holding your pee until you find an appropriate place to squat. You can do it through Kegel exercises, where you squeeze the muscles repeatedly several times a day. Try squeezing 10 times in a row, five times daily. If you're not sure which muscles to squeeze, try stopping yourself from peeing after you've started. You stop the flow using your PC muscles.

If doing exercise sounds too hard, you can take the easy way and use Ben Wa balls for about 10 minutes a day.

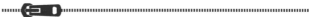

Desperate Times, *Desperate Measures*

66 I have to admit, I once refused to use an outhouse on Vancouver Island that was extremely foul. Dirty, stinky, with flies everywhere. I had to pee very badly, so I opted instead to go into the ice-cold Pacific Ocean with my shorts on, and did it there. I was one of the very few people in the water. My fellow campers were astonished that I went in, but they didn't know I had a good reason! **99**

—MM

These two small, heavy balls are worn inside your vagina, forcing you to contract the muscles to keep them from dropping out. Or you can try "love balls," which are connected with a string, kind of like a tampon, and inserted into the vagina. "They're passive, so you can just leave them in all day, and you're strengthening the muscles without even thinking about it," explains Nicola Mercer, director of d.vice designer sex gear. "It only takes two or three weeks to have pelvic muscles of steel."

Not only are the pelvic floor muscles important for bladder control, but being able to tighten them on command can also be a big plus during sex. But we'll get into that more in a couple of chapters.

For paddlers, the peeing problems are a bit different. You can use the methods mentioned earlier once you pull off the water and head into the wilderness, but if you're paddling for several hours at a time, you may need to relieve yourself before you stop. "If it will be a long way between take-outs, women don't have the option of 'pumping the bilges' directly over the side as men can," says Philip Torrens of MEC. He has this suggestion: "Cut the top off a plastic bleach bottle on the diagonal (keep the screw cap on it). This will make a form-fitting relief reservoir that can double as a bailing scoop for the canoe."

Dealing with Your Period

Camping with your period is no big deal, but it does require planning. If your period is unpredictable, make sure you are prepared to get it while camping. You can't stop and buy a box of tampons once you're in the middle of the forest.

Some women would rather not deal with their periods at all while they're camping, so they schedule camping trips between cycles. Women who take birth control pills also have the option of skipping a period if it's going to coincide with camping plans by ignoring the placebos that make up the fourth week of the pack and starting a new pack right away. It's an easy and effective choice, but it can lead to breakthrough bleeding at other times if you do it too often.

If you decide to let nature take its course, getting your period during a camping trip is no problem for most women. For paddlers, it's easier to use tampons so you can jump into the water whenever you want without worrying about soggy pads. A lot of backpackers also prefer tampons since they are smaller to carry and can be burned in a campfire if necessary. It's best to pack used tampons out with your other trash. Never bury them in the woods because the smell of blood may attract curious animals that will dig them up and make a mess. Nobody wants to see your shredded, used tampons all over a hiking trail or campsite.

Pads are a little tougher to deal with because most of them have a plastic backing. This means that they aren't biodegradable, even after a long time, and shouldn't be disposed of in a fire, either. If you use pads while camping in the backcountry, you'll have to keep the used ones in a trash bag and throw them away when you get back to civilization. The same goes for plastic tampon applicators.

There is some debate about whether bears are attracted to the smell of menstrual blood. Actually, it's one of the reasons that a lot of women try to avoid camping when they're having their period. Still, there's no conclusive evidence about this. If you prefer to err on the side of caution, you can reduce the scent of used pads or tampons by sprinkling crushed aspirins on them and wrapping them in foil before you put them in the plastic trash bag. Many women just use a double bag to reduce the scent. You should always hang the bag with your other garbage away from your tent if you are taking bear precautions.

A third option for taking care of your period is gaining some popularity among women campers. A small, rubber or silicone cup can be worn internally to hold the blood, and cleaned out a couple of times per day. These cups are specially designed for this purpose and sold under a number of brand names, including the Keeper, DivaCup, and Mooncup. If you use one of these, there's no need to dispose of any waste, or to carry it out with you. While the cup should be washed whenever you empty it, you can just give it a wipe with a tissue for the time being, and continue to wear it until you reach an easier place to wash it properly. They can take some getting used to, so don't try it for the first time on a camping trip. Try your cup at home for a month or two, then decide if you want to take it camping.

If you get bad cramps with your period, keep a supply of your favorite medication in your first-aid kit. You probably won't be able to lie around in a fetal position all day, so you're better off if you can keep the cramps under control with pills.

Other Nasty Business

The last thing you want to deal with on a camping trip is a yeast or a bladder infection. It's irritating when you get these things at home, but in the middle of the woods, it's enough to make you want to call the whole thing off.

If you are prone to yeast infections, make sure you have your regular treatment in your first-aid kit. If you're going to be away for more than a night or two, it's worth the extra precaution. Also pack extra pairs of underpants.

Wearing dirty, sweaty panties can increase your likelihood of an infection. If you're trying to pack light, try using a fresh panty liner every day instead. It's the next best thing to clean underpants.

Bladder infections, also known as urinary tract infections, can make it nearly unbearable to be camping. You constantly have to stop for a pee break, and you feel terrible. If you get bladder infections, take whatever precautions you can while you're out camping. The most important thing to do is drink a lot of water. This will flush any bacteria out of your system as you go. Trying not to pee for hours on end will make things worse, so stop for pee breaks whenever you feel the urge.

Cranberries are a popular, natural treatment for bladder infections, but obviously you can't walk around with gallons of cranberry juice, just in case. A lot of vitamin and herbal remedy companies now produce cranberry capsules that are potent and much easier to carry. If you get infections from time to time, make them part of your first-aid kit. The other option is to ask your doctor for an antibiotics prescription that will cure a bladder infection, and bring the pills with you just in case. If you do this, keep an eye on the expiry date.

If you're camping with guys, they may tell you that you are bringing along a lot of unnecessary stuff. Tampons when you don't have your period, yeast-infection treatments, panty liners, cranberry pills—all of it might seem crazy to a guy. But if you do get your period or an infection, it will make life horrible for you if you don't have these items. I'll give the final word on the matter to Nikki, who gave me this advice: "Don't let the boy see what you are packing, because it is all essential!"

Chapter 4:

CREATING A ROMANTIC DINNER

from a Ziploc Bag

My boyfriend, Gerhard, looks at food and sees the fuel he needs to carry on with his day. I look at food and see a reason to live! Food, for people like me, is a highly sensual pleasure. Yes, we need it to live, but there's so much more to it than that. In fact, the preparation and eating of food is one of the few things in life that involves all of our senses. (And as its lusty relationship with eating may suggest, sex is another.)

Taste may be the first thing that comes to mind when you think of eating, but every other sense combines with that one to make the experience complete. If you read the words "freshly baked bread" or "popcorn," you are more likely to think of their scent than their taste. Smell is incredibly powerful, and can change our moods instantly. Indeed, certain food scents have been connected to our libido as well. Licorice, cinnamon, and orange are all smells that are said to make us feel more turned on.

The sight of food affects us, too. The plume of steam rising from a bowl of oatmeal in the morning gives us comfort, while the rich darkness of a fudge brownie promises a decadent experience to match.

Touch is not the first thing you'd think of when it comes to food, but the softness of bread in your mouth, and the satisfying crunch of an apple are highly sensual experiences. Using our hands to eat increases those sensual moments. Doesn't honey taste better when you're licking it off your fingers, or, better yet, someone else's fingers?

Even our hearing has a part to play in whetting our appetites. Who wouldn't be tempted out of their sleeping bag in the morning by the sound of bacon sizzling in a frying pan? By engaging all of our senses, food can bring out our desires and fulfill us in a way that can only be matched by the sense of satisfaction we get from devouring a lover.

As you can see, food gives me enormous pleasure, and never more than when I'm camping. My senses are already heightened by the sun warming my skin while the wind simultaneously cools it. My breathing is deeper from the fresh air mixed with exercise. The sounds of moving water and nearby wildlife fill my ears. With all senses alive, I'm ready to joyfully embrace the experience of eating.

Gerhard, on the other hand, would be perfectly happy just to add up calories and make sure he's getting enough—or so he says. But when we reach the end of our day and set up camp, the first thing he wants is a warm drink or a mug of soup. Clearly, he has sensual cravings for liquid heat, even if he doesn't realize it.

Food is a wonderful motivator. It can affect our moods in all kinds of ways, good and bad. So when you plan out your meals for a camping trip, you are also planning out your moods. Since our goal is to set a romantic and sexy mood, I'm going to concentrate on romantic recipes to add to your camping repertoire. (For a more complete range of recipes, see the camping cookbooks listed in Appendix 3 at the end of the book.)

Car camping offers almost unlimited possibilities for cooking since you can bring along a cooler with perishable foods. And for those trips, you can find a favorite recipe in a cookbook to take with you. But to be fair to everyone, all of the recipes here are suitable for paddlers as well as backpackers, who have to be worried about foods going off or taking up too much space. All of these recipes are for two generous servings. So if you're camping with a group, you'll need to increase the quantities.

If you're paddling aggressively, backpacking up a steep route, or steaming up the tent, you'll need to eat up to twice what you normally do, and even more for cold-weather trips. But your needs are based on your size, and you'll want to think about that before splitting your gourmet dinner in half with your partner. (This is where my boyfriend's mathematical approach to eating is not without its uses.) If one of you weighs 30 percent more than the other, that person needs about 30 percent more food to keep going. For active trips, count on chowing down on at least 2800 calories per day for the average woman, and at least 3500 calories for the average man.

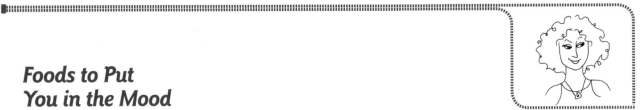

Foods to Put You in the Mood

Throughout history (and throughout my own experience), certain foods have acted as aphrodisiacs, leading to nights of passion. The properties that make these foods crank up your libido are mysterious, even magical. But there's no doubt that food can make us feel sexier. If you're looking to spice up your next trip, here are some foods I recommend:

LICORICE:
The scent is a sexual stimulant, especially for men. And its chewy texture elicits a craving to nibble on just about anything. (Just make sure it's all out of your teeth before you flash a smile, or you might ruin the effect!)

STRAWBERRIES:
Ever notice how a well-formed strawberry looks like the head of a penis? What man could help but be turned on watching his lover thoroughly enjoy a rich, ripe strawberry?

CINNAMON:
This one is more about scent than anything else, so eat something that will give you cinnamon breath, or bake some fresh cinnamon bannock and let the smell waft. If the cinnamon is spicy enough, it'll warm you up so much, you'll need to share the heat.

COUSCOUS:
Traditionally, this Moroccan dish is eaten with your fingers, which puts you in a sensual mood, ready for other tantalizing sensations.

"SPIKED" HOT CHOCOLATE:
I needn't go into detail for the women. Chocolate has an unmatched ability to boost your mood. This warm, sweet drink makes you feel relaxed and secure, while a bit of alcohol gets rid of any lingering inhibitions.

NUTS:
Nuts contain essential fatty acids that help keep your hormone levels up. And you were going to bring them anyway, right?

HONEY:
Go for the direct approach and lick it off each other. It's the perfect way to entice your lover to give you an enthusiastic blow job.

MULLED WINE:
Some inexpensive red wine and mulling spices can turn up the heat on a cold night. Just don't overdo it, or you'll start to get more sleepy than horny.

OYSTERS:
The classic prelude to love! If you're lucky enough to be camping near a source of fresh, raw oysters, you can get the traditional experience; otherwise, the smoked version will have to do.

DARK CHOCOLATE:
Chocolate is powerful enough to mention twice. Eating high-quality dark chocolate releases the same chemical in our brains that gets released when we fall in love. Need I say more?

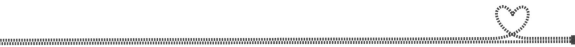

Breakfast: Refueling After a Big Night

For Wisconsin native Barbara, breakfast is a good time to get that first cuddle of the day. She and her boyfriend always make up a big pot of porridge, and huddle together in the morning chill dipping their spoons into it. "For some reason, I always feel like it's terribly romantic to eat out of the same dish," she says. "There's something about it that just makes us feel really close at those moments. Sharing food is like sharing breath. It's something you need for your basic survival." (On the practical side, this burst of morning romance also means they have only one bowl to clean.)

Val told me she finds comfort in the sounds of making breakfast at camp. "I love the ritual of my little gas stove's hiss in the morning when boiling water for coffee," she says.

Breakfast is your first activity of the day, and it can help to set the mood. On a cold morning, eating your breakfast inside the tent while still huddling in your sleeping bags can feel as decadent as room service at a fancy hotel. The smell of fresh coffee is like a signal to your senses that a new day has begun.

At home, many of us skip breakfast, or grab something on the go. But if you're going to be active all day (and if you've had a little nighttime activity), you need to get your energy reserves loaded up after 12 hours or so of not eating. And breakfast doesn't have to be the same, boring instant oatmeal or cold granola every time you go camping.

Egg-based breakfasts are popular with car campers, but few backpackers and paddlers are willing to risk the mess of broken eggs in their gear. You can buy a small plastic egg carrier at most camping shops that helps to increase your odds of transporting the goods without any breakage. Another option is to buy a carton of egg replacement and freeze it solid. If you pack it frozen, it will stay cold overnight and your first breakfast on the trail can be lovely scrambled eggs or an omelet, or bring some extra bread along and make French toast.

Recipes on pages 68–70.

Lunch: Keep It Simple to Keep Going

Lana and Greg are one of those "hiking club marriages." There's quite a history of them at their hiking club in Southern Ontario. Not surprisingly, many of these romances began over a meal—shared outside. Lana and Greg met at one of their club's social nights, and Greg asked Lana if she wanted to go hiking with him. "I wasn't sure if it was supposed to be a date or not, but I decided I'd make it into one," Lana recalls.

The best way to turn a run-of-the-mill hike into a date? A romantic picnic lunch! "I told him I'd take care of lunch, and I packed a bottle of wine, and sandwiches on fresh, crusty bread with marinated veggies and cheese,"

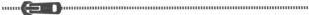

You Can't Trust a Man to Shop

66 I met my boyfriend through a social club for singles, so we did quite a bit of camping together before we were even dating, but it was always with a group. We'd have a leader organizing the whole thing and telling us what to bring. But after we started seeing each other, we thought it might be nice to get away without the group around—just the two of us. We'd been on enough trips that we figured we knew what we needed.

The first time we planned a camping trip alone, I was really busy at work, so he offered to buy the food. When we got there, I found out that our food for the next four days consisted of granola, energy bars, peanuts, peanut butter, a loaf of bread (smushed in his pack), and two-minute noodles. I nearly killed him! After that, I started making a shopping list for every trip, or went to get the food myself. It would have been bearable if he'd at least remembered to get some chocolate! 99

—MN

Lana says. "For dessert, we had fresh strawberries and chocolate dipping sauce. It weighed a ton, but I think it made the right impression."

It must have—after they returned home, they met up again in the evening...and then again for many more hikes, lunches, and evenings. "Eventually," Lana says, "we got married. Our wedding cake had a bride-and-groom pair of moose on top. The female one even had a little veil."

Many first dates among outdoorsy couples take place outside—on a hike, at a ski hill, in a mountain bike park, or maybe down a river, if the two are paddlers. Lana had a surefire way to convince Greg that theirs was a date. I had a similar experience where my date brought a gourmet picnic, complete with wine, to our first outing at the zoo.

Even if your relationship is well-established, lunchtime can be a wonderful opportunity to keep the romance fresh. Lunch is a great time to surprise your partner with expressions of love. If you're putting together the lunch ingredients for the day, sneak in a little treat that your partner isn't expecting. It could be his or her favorite kind of cookie or candy bar. Perhaps it's a juice box to break up the monotony of lukewarm water. How about a decadent fudge brownie? If you don't want to pack extra food to surprise your partner, you can sneak a little love note into his or her lunch instead. Whatever will put a smile on your faces and get you going again is a good idea.

If the weather is particularly harsh and you've managed to find a sheltered place to stop for lunch, it may be worth the extra time and effort to have something warm. A cup of tea or soup can make a huge difference if you've been cold and wet all morning. It will warm you up from the inside out, and put you both in a much better mood.

Most of the time, camping lunches are served on the go. Most campers find a place to stop for a rest and put together a quick bite that takes little or no preparation. Unfortunately, that can lead to boring, repetitive lunches

full of peanut butter sandwiches, or salami and cheese. In general, flat breads like pita pockets, tortilla wraps, or crackers travel better than regular bread. If you're on a long trip, bring a couple of different options so you don't eat the same kind of lunch every day. A little bit of creativity can make lunch a lot more enjoyable.

Rather than thinking of lunch as a purely functional necessity, try to look at it as a lovely picnic opportunity. Find a scenic place to stop and enjoy your lunch where the view is to die for, or you are serenaded by the cheerful babble of a stream. Or go farther from the beaten track so that you can make out a little when you're done with lunch. Spread your jackets out on the ground and settle in for a snuggle.

Recipes on pages 70–71.

Snacks: Beyond Trail Mix

What could be better to rejuvenate you on the trail than GORP—good old raisins and peanuts? Quite a lot of things, actually! When you're out being active all day, snacks are essential for keeping your energy up between meals. The two things you're usually trying to replace by snacking are your used-up calories (energy) and your sweated-out salt. But there's no reason why snacks have to be repetitive and functional. Snacking is when you can be wonderfully indulgent. Don't just stop to fill up your empty stomach—make it a moment of pleasure in your day. Include flavors that really turn you on. Spice things up, or make them lick-your-lips salty. Here are some suggestions that will get you out of your trail-mix routine while replenishing your all-important salt levels:

– Hickory-smoked almonds: They're lower in fat than peanuts and even contain calcium to make up for the milk you probably aren't drinking while you camp.

– Pistachios: Buy the ones with white shells so you don't stain your fingers red.

– Beef or salmon jerky

– Mini papadums

– Flavored snack crackers: BBQ and cheese flavors have lots of salt.

– Bits 'n bites: Mix your favorite cereal or crackers for a salty treat.

– Rice cracker mix/Oriental mix

– CornNuts

As anyone who has ever "swallowed" knows, a man's ejaculate can be quite salty. Of course, you'll have to find somewhere private to have it as a snack food, and while one of you is getting your salt level restored, the other is having it depleted. If you're both men, you can even things out, but if your woman is making a salty treat of

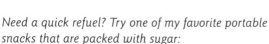

Energy Boosters

Need a quick refuel? Try one of my favorite portable snacks that are packed with sugar:

Tropical fruit salad: Dried mango, papaya, and pineapple

Yogurt-dipped raisins: Also try yogurt-dipped peanuts and cranberries.

Ferrero Rocher chocolates or any individually wrapped chocolate

Fig Newtons: Or try date or raspberry cookies.

Licorice, all sorts

Peanut brittle

Fudge

Chocolate-covered coffee beans: The ultimate pick-me-up!

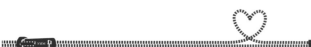

you, you'll just have to find another way to replenish your supplies. Still, you get a blow job and she gets salt (and protein), so it's a win-win!

Chocolate is probably the most universally loved treat for campers. It provides both an energy hit and a psychological boost that revives even the most exhausted of us. In fact, for many campers, chocolate is not a treat—it's a necessity!

Philip Torrens of Mountain Equipment Co-op learned the hard way to take his wife's chocolate needs seriously. "On the first camping trip my now-wife and I did together, she asked me to bring chocolate," he says. "I naively chucked a single bar into the food bag. That got gobbled the first evening. The next day, she was looking for more. We damn near broke up over that."

Now she's in charge of the chocolate supply, even though Torrens organizes all of the other food. That way, it's up to his wife to make sure they don't run out. (Sometimes you have to leave it to the expert.) Torrens also suggests carrying your chocolate in a sealed plastic bag in bear country to reduce odors. But he adds, "I think it would be a very sorry bear that tried to take the chocolate cache away from my wife."

If you're stopping for a snack break anyway, why not make it a romance break, too? You can find a secluded place for a cuddle and a smooch, or maybe even more. To make sure you have the energy for an extra romp, start off with some sexy treats. Individually wrapped chocolate peppermint patties or after-dinner mints will freshen up your breath to make you more kissable, as will cinnamon hearts. The scent of licorice can arouse desire, so take a few pieces along with you and make yourself irresistible. Once you've taken a moment to satisfy your hunger, you can focus on your more intimate needs!

Dinner: Romantic Meals in a Baggie or Two

Sadly, the most romantic dinner location I've ever visited was wasted on a group trip when I was single. I sat with my hot, fragrant plate of chicken and pasta, watching the sun splash its last, golden rays over the breathtaking vistas of the Grand Canyon. Our campsite was perched on the Canyon's edge, providing million-dollar views. A gentle breeze made me forget the desert heat. The exhausting day slipped effortlessly into the past. If any man on that trip had made a move on me that night, I would have been his.

Adding romance to your outdoor dining is easy to do, given the wonderful scenery most campers enjoy. Just being out in the wild, in a quiet setting is a good start. Having a nice view where you choose to eat is also going to add to the romance. If you can, arrange your "dinner table" so you can watch the sunset together. Sunsets bring out almost everyone's romantic side.

If you're near a lake, river, or coast, sit down to eat with a view of the water. Nothing is sexier than the sound of crashing waves or rushing rapids. And if there are mountains in the distance, make those your backdrop and soak up the majesty. Sit yourselves nice and close to each other, thighs touching. Dinner time is usually more leisurely than other meal breaks, since you've got no-where to run off to afterward—so make yourselves really comfortable and enjoy the scenery that you've worked so hard to reach.

The romance doesn't have to end when the sun has gone down. You can enjoy a private, candlelight dinner in the wilderness. Could anything be better? Sit close together and watch the flickering light on your partner's face. Everyone looks sexier by the soft light of a candle, so try to tear your eyes away from your food now and then and make eye contact. The more your partner sees you staring, the clearer the signal you're sending—I think you're hot, and I'm going to show you how I feel as soon as we finish eating!

Tea candles are small and light and can add some class to any evening. They are a particularly nice addition if you're not going to have a campfire. Citronella candles

can help to keep the bugs at bay while they light the way to passion. The Body Shop also makes special travel candles that come in a tin with a lid for multinight use.

Drinks: High Country Happy Hour

If you're car camping, it's easy to bring along a bottle or two of wine to make the evening complete. Carrying glass bottles in a backpack or canoe is a bit risky (and heavy!), so it's good to get a little more creative if you'd like to drink alcohol during your backcountry trip. If you're not offended by the idea, you can pour your wine into a plastic water bottle, or a wine skin (go figure.) There's something delightfully naughty about drinking wine out of your camping mug.

Val likes to go for the high-class approach. "I always take silver-plated goblets along," she says. "They don't break when they fall over, and they look infinitely more festive and elegant." Sure, but can you trust the raccoons not to run off with them? If you're a little short on silver goblets, most camping stores carry Lexan wine and cocktail glasses that look almost as nice as glass but won't break. You can even get champagne flutes for those special occasions.

Beer can be brought along in cans, as long as you don't shake it up too badly. The biggest challenge with beer is keeping it cold, so paddlers often put it in a bag and tie it to the canoe or kayak so they can chill their brewskies in the water.

Almost anything non-carbonated can be brought along in a plastic bottle—whiskey, sherry, port, or your favorite liqueur. Whatever you like to share, having a little something to drink during or after dinner can make the day's efforts fade away and prepare you for a night of togetherness.

On chilly nights, you can add an ounce or two of liqueur to a cup of hot cocoa. Peppermint schnapps is great for this, as are Kahlua and Frangelico. If you're not a drinker, then cocoa can always benefit from a few marshmallows.

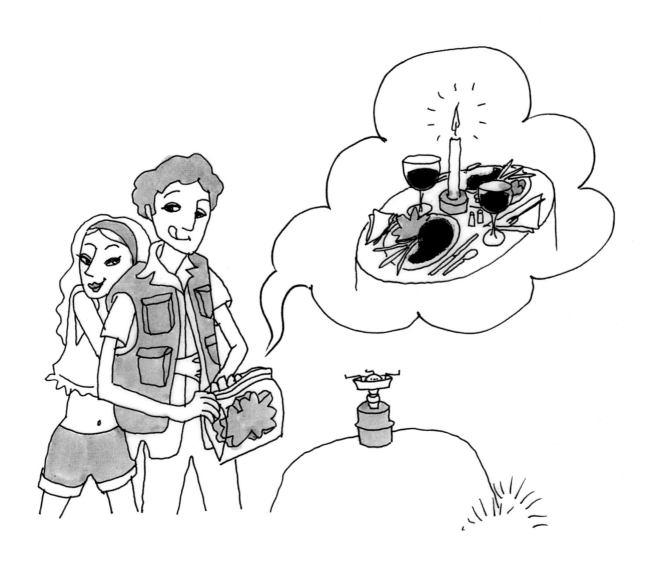

Coffee with Irish cream is another warm evening treat, and the extra shot of caffeine at the end of the day will perk you up for a passionate night together.

Outdoor Hors D'oeuvres

Just because you're roughing it doesn't mean a three-course meal is out of the question. If you are getting hungry but dinner is going to take a while to prepare, there are some nice appetizers you can have on hand to stop your tummy from grumbling. There's a popular theory among men that a woman is comfortable with herself (and therefore not "high maintenance") if she orders an appetizer when you're out for dinner. This is the backwoods equivalent—so ladies, don't be shy about spoiling your appetite. I'm sure you will both find a way to work off the extra calories!

By keeping a few extra ingredients around, you'll always be ready to have a gourmet lead-up to your dinner.

Recipes on pages 72–73.

Enchanting Entrees

The entree is the main event when it comes to dinner. Now is the time to have something that really turns on your taste buds after a day of hard work. You're not in a hurry, so you can savor every bite. You don't need a big kitchen or a lot of electric appliances to make a delicious meal. You just need a few well-chosen ingredients and a tiny stove with a couple of pots. I've always believed that food tastes better when you eat it outside, so you've already got an advantage over your regular meals. Try some of the delectable dinners for two in this chapter, and banish the instant ramen noodles from your camping trips forever.

Many of the recipes in this chapter require powdered sauce mixes that are available at most supermarkets. I haven't specified brand names because availability is so different from place to place. When you shop for your trip, make sure you look at the directions for the sauce.

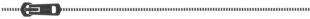

The Dinner *that Got Away*

66 We were backpacking in Arizona, and we brought along some meat to put in our first dinner. It would have spoiled very quickly left out in the intense heat, but the river beside our campsite was nice and cool. So we put the baggie of meat into a mesh bag and tied it to a rock so that the meat was sitting in the cold water, along with the beers my boyfriend had insisted on hauling out there with us.

A few hours later, when we were ready to make dinner, I pulled the bag out of the river. Some kind of fish had found our meat and chewed right through the baggie to eat it! After a long day of hiking in the desert heat, we had only bread, potatoes, and cheese for dinner. But at least the beers were cold. 99

—JS

If it requires milk, you'll have to buy some powdered milk to bring with you for backpacking and paddling trips.

There are also dehydrated ingredients listed. If you have the space (or strength) to bring fresh ingredients instead, I encourage it. Fresh veggies should last for at least two days before they start to get mushy. If not, some stores sell dehydrated veggies and TVP (textured vegetable protein), or you can dehydrate your own foods in your oven by spreading them on a cookie sheet in a single layer and putting them in the oven on the lowest temperature setting for several hours. Dehydrators, which will help speed up the process, are available in some camping shops. Whatever method you use, be sure to dehydrate the ingredients completely. If there is any moisture left, they could get moldy over time.

The recipes in this chapter won't just fill the void, they'll satisfy you with sophisticated flavors and wonderful

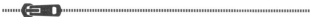

I Dream of
Betty Crocker

66 I love watching my wife cook. I don't know why, but I find it really sexy—all of that chopping, beating, and stirring. She's so in control when she's making food, like the conductor of an orchestra who knows what she wants every single instrument to do and how to make it happen.

At home, I can steal glances from the living room, and she doesn't realize I'm watching her. But when we're out camping and she's sitting on a rock, stirring the pot and adding spices, I sometimes can't resist coming up behind her and nuzzling her neck. She always acts all annoyed at me, like I'm interrupting her careful work, but she can't help giggling whenever I do it. And then she has a cute little grin on her face for the next 10 minutes.

I can completely see why women find it sexy when a man cooks for them. I should really learn how, but I'm having too much fun watching her do it. **99**

—RM

textures. A delicious, gourmet dinner will make the evening feel like more like a date than a survival challenge. Once your romantic date in the wilderness progresses past dinner, there are sure to be more physical delights ahead!

Recipes on pages 73–76.

Sounds Fishy to Me

Serving up a fresh fish that you've caught yourself is one of the most satisfying things to do for a camping dinner. It harkens right back to our hunter/gatherer past, giving you the sense that you are a provider at the most basic level. Time to live out your caveman fantasies! Plus, fresh fish prepared over a fire is delicious.

If you are planning to fish on your trip, bring along some herbs and spices to flavor your catch. Rosemary and thyme are both nice on fish, or a bit of dried dill. A pinch of dried lemon zest will add immeasurably to the flavor. Fresh fish is so succulent that it would be a crime to drown it in sauce, so just sprinkle on your herbs of choice and throw it in a pan with a little oil. When the flesh is opaque and flaky, it's ready to eat.

A camping trip to Vancouver Island gave Tasha and her husband a rare chance to buy live crab straight from the fishermen. When they reached their campsite for the night, they were all ready to make a romantic seafood dinner. Tasha was getting the rest of dinner ready while her husband dealt with the crabs.

"He held up the crab in front of him before dropping him in the water and exclaimed, 'Ha! You're just a big bug!'" Tasha recalls. "At which point, the crab clamped down on his finger. Hard." This was followed by a lot of screaming as her husband tried to fling the crab off his hand. "He danced around with it clamped down on him for a very long half minute until the 'bug' finally let go," she says. "Then we managed to wrestle it into the pot. My husband had a seriously bruised finger, but the crab definitely got the worst of the deal, because we ate him for dinner and he was delicious!"

I suppose there's a lesson in there about not playing with your food. Fresh shellfish are a bit hard to gather for yourself without specialized fishing equipment or diving gear, but if you're lucky enough to get some, it does cook up nicely by just boiling it. If you think you might have that opportunity, bring a lemon to squeeze over the seafood and bring out all of the lovely, fresh flavor.

It's in the Bag

For lightweight backpackers or people on long paddling trips, freezer-bag cooking is gaining popularity. This method involves using only dehydrated and instant foods, supplemented with pouches or cans of meat or tofu. The idea is to put all of the dry ingredients for a meal into one heavy-duty freezer bag, and then boil water using a kettle or pot. Measure off some water with a plastic cup, pour it directly into the freezer bag, and then mix it with a plastic spoon. No pointy tools can be used because they might poke through the bag. Wait a few minutes for everything to rehydrate, add your pouch or can of meat if needed, and dinner can be eaten right out of the bag.

The advantages of this method are that everything is prepared very quickly and simply, and there are no dishes to clean, except your spoons. You have to carry only one pot to boil water. The meals are generally very light to carry, and you can bring a variety of individual dinners so you don't have to eat the same meal as your partner if you don't feel like it. This is a great way to keep the peace if the two of you just don't like the same foods.

The main drawback is the preparation time involved before your trip. Everything must be precooked and dehydrated, including pasta. If you think this method is for you, you'll need a dehydrator. To find out more about freezer-bag cooking, check out this helpful website: www.freezerbagcooking.com.

Don't Forget Dessert

Any meal or snack can be romantic, but somehow dessert is the sexiest of all. Maybe it's because we eat dessert closer to when we'll be in bed, or perhaps it's just the great sugar rush that heightens our lust. Dessert is all about pure pleasure, and what could be naughtier than that?

Florida paddler Craig discovered a side of his fiancee he'd never seen before when they started camping together. Their first trip was a big letdown for her, because a fire ban prevented them from toasting marshmallows. This, apparently, was what camping was all about for her.

"The next time, she made me check ahead on the conditions, or she wouldn't even want to go," he says. But there had been enough rain to allow campfires again, so their first night out he built his very best fire. "By the time we finished dinner, there were some great coals at the base of the fire—perfect toasting conditions!" Craig remembers. "She was in a playful mood, or maybe the sugar was getting to her, and she put a marshmallow in her mouth and kissed me, oozing the marshmallow into my mouth with her tongue." He returned the favor, and soon they found themselves licking and sucking gooey marshmallow off each other. "We ended up spreading out the blanket we were sitting on, and having sex right in front of the fire," he says. Who knew a bit of sugar could be so hot?

With or without a campfire, there are plenty of treats you can easily bring along on a camping trip for a sweet end to your dinner. Cookies are one of the easiest and most likely to survive the trip. Brownies are also pretty resilient, particularly the ones without frosting. Of course, as Craig knows, toasted marshmallows are a classic, and you can bring along graham crackers and chocolate to make s'mores. Let's face it, we never grow out of some things!

There are a huge variety of instant puddings, pies, and cheesecake mixes available that you can whip up after dinner, too. If you're trying to make the occasion even more special, make one of the dessert recipes I've included in this chapter. They're all decadent and sexy, and sure to put you both in the mood to get a little skin-on-skin exercise.

Recipes on pages 76–77.

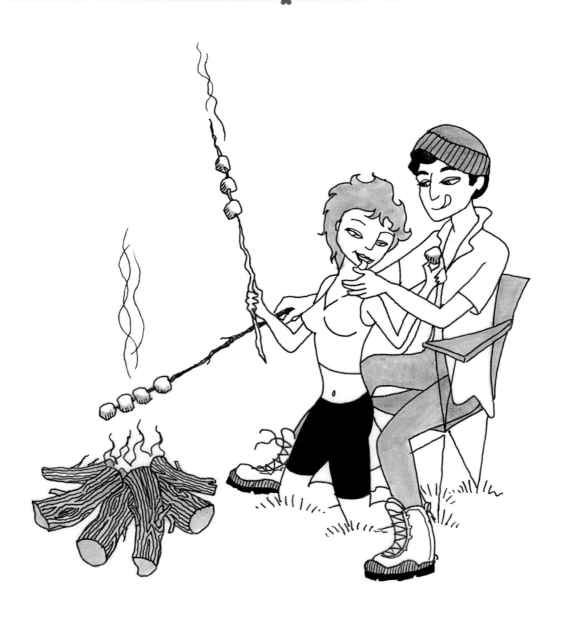

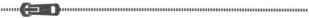

Sample Menu for a Fabulously **Romantic Camping Weekend**

Let's assume that your trip begins with your arrival at a campsite on Friday evening and continues until dinner time on Sunday. When you plan out a menu so that you never eat the same thing twice, it shows that you are making a real effort to make every meal special. If you want to make your partner fall in love with you—and camping—all over again, follow this menu of indulgent delights.

FRIDAY
Dinner: Smoked Chicken Alfredo with Mushrooms, white wine

Dessert: Spiked Strawberry Shortcake with fresh berries, mixed berry herbal tea

SATURDAY
Breakfast: "Whatever You Like" Omelette, coffee

Morning Snacks: Tropical fruit salad, hickory-smoked almonds

Lunch: Round-the-World Cheese Sandwiches

Afternoon Snacks: Ferrero Rocher chocolates, mini papadums

Hors D'oeuvres: Crackers with smoked oysters and chili sauce

Dinner: Malaysian Satay Tofu, red wine

Dessert: Sex in a Pan, hot chocolate with Kahlua

SUNDAY
Breakfast: Chocolate-Chip Pancakes, coffee

Morning Snacks: Pistachios, yogurt-dipped cranberries

Lunch: Hide the Salami (in a Sandwich)

Afternoon Snacks: Chocolate-covered coffee beans, salmon jerky

Hors D'oeuvres: Mediterranean Passion Pitas

Dinner: Cheesy Chicken Quesadillas

Dessert: Sinful Chocolate Fondue, peppermint tea

Chocolate-Chip Pancakes

Serves 2

Whoever decided that it was okay to have chocolate for breakfast deserves a medal!

INGREDIENTS:
Instant pancake mix, prepared to package directions for two servings

1 tbsp. oil or margarine

$\frac{1}{2}$ cup chocolate chips

Alternatives to chocolate chips: $\frac{1}{2}$ cup dried blueberries, strawberries, cherries, or cranberries soaked in $\frac{1}{2}$ cup hot water for two minutes

$\frac{1}{4}$ cup maple syrup

INSTRUCTIONS:
Heat oil or margarine in a frying pan over a medium flame. Prepare pancake batter according to the directions. Stir in chocolate chips. Pour dollops of batter into the frying pan to make pancakes roughly the size of an open hand. When the bottoms are golden brown and bubbles form on the tops, flip the pancakes over. When golden brown on both sides, the pancakes are ready. Serve with maple syrup.

The "Whatever You Like" Omelette

Serves 2

INGREDIENTS:

4 eggs or equivalent in egg substitute

2 tbsp. cold water

1 tbsp. olive oil

½ tsp. dehydrated garlic or garlic powder

Salt and pepper to taste

Dried onion flakes (optional)

Dehydrated mushrooms, soaked in hot water for one minute (optional)

Dehydrated red or green peppers, soaked in hot water for one minute (optional)

Sun-dried tomatoes, soaked in hot water for three minutes, then sliced (optional)

Sliced olives packed in a small baggie or plastic container (optional)

½ cup shredded cheese (cheddar, colby, mozzarella, gruyere, or Swiss)

INSTRUCTIONS:

Heat olive oil in a large frying pan over a medium flame. In a bowl or pot, beat the eggs together with the water, garlic, salt, and pepper, plus whatever optional ingredients you have brought. Pour the egg mixture into the frying pan and cook until the top is wet but not runny. Loosen the omelette by carefully sliding a spatula under the edges, working your way around the pan. Flip the omelette over carefully using the spatula, or, if you're feeling lucky, toss it up and catch it in the pan. Sprinkle the shredded cheese over the omelette and continue to cook for one minute. Fold the omelette in half, then cut into two servings. Serve with bread or pitas if you have an active day ahead.

Super-Easy Rice Pudding

Serves 2

Rice pudding for breakfast? Why not! It's yummy and gives you all of those carbs you need to get moving.

INGREDIENTS:

1 cup water

1 cup instant rice

½ package instant vanilla pudding (prepared to package directions)

½ cup raisins

1 tsp. cinnamon

INSTRUCTIONS:

Boil the water and add rice. Remove from heat, cover, and let stand for 5 minutes. Meanwhile, make the instant pudding according to the directions. Add the pudding, raisins and cinnamon to the rice and mix thoroughly.

Breakfast Couscous

Serves 2

INGREDIENTS:

I cup water

I tsp. oil or margarine

I cup instant couscous

6 dried apricots, cut into small chunks

¼ cup dried currants or raisins

½ cup sliced almonds

I tsp. cinnamon

2 tbsp. sugar (or to taste)

INSTRUCTIONS:

Boil the water with the oil or margarine. Remove from heat, add the couscous, dried apricots, and currants (or raisins). Stir and cover. Let stand for five minutes. Stir in sugar, cinnamon, and almonds and serve hot.

Round-the-World Cheese Sandwiches

Serves 2

INGREDIENTS:

6 slices mild cheese (cheddar, colby, mozzarella, or havarti)

2 large pita pockets

INSTRUCTIONS:

Add 3 slices of cheese to each pita pocket, then finish off with one of the following combinations:

* Italian: I pinch each of basil and oregano, plus 2 tsp. tomato paste (can be bought in tubes with screw-on lids)

* Mexican: I pinch of cumin and I fast-food packet of salsa

* Greek: I pinch of rubbed rosemary, plus a few olive slices

* Thanksgiving Special: 2 tbsp. dried cranberries and I tbsp. apple butter (or apple sauce)

Thai Peanut Butter Wraps

Serves 2

INGREDIENTS:

4 small or 2 large tortilla wraps

4 tbsp. peanut butter (preferably without added sugar)

¼ tsp. powdered ginger

1 fast-food packet of chili sauce (get extras when you order Chinese take-out)

½ cup fresh alfalfa sprouts or bean sprouts (optional)

INSTRUCTIONS:

Spread peanut butter on the tortilla wraps. Top with a little chili sauce, and sprinkle on a pinch of ginger. Place the sprouts in the middle of each wrap, then fold up the bottom about 2 inches and roll up the wrap from one side.

Hide the Salami (in a Sandwich)

Serves 2

INGREDIENTS:

10 slices of your favorite salami

2 large pita pockets

2 fast-food packets of mustard (from your local deli or burger joint)

½ small cucumber

4 slices provolone or mozzarella cheese (optional)

INSTRUCTIONS:

Spread the mustard around the insides of the pita pockets. Arrange the salami (and cheese) slices in the pockets. Slice the cucumber and add to the pockets.

Camping Canapes

Serves 2

INGREDIENTS:
12 small crackers (plain, not flavored)

INSTRUCTIONS:
Top with one of the following combinations:

– 12 smoked oysters and a packet of take-out hot sauce

– 6 oz. of canned crab and 12 cucumber slices

– 12 small slices mozzarella cheese and 12 sun-dried tomatoes (soak the tomatoes in hot water for five minutes first)

Muchas Mexican Heat

INGREDIENTS:

½ package instant black bean dip mix

Water as required from dip mix package directions

6 packets of take-out salsa

1 tbsp. fresh coriander leaves, chopped (optional)

Plain, chili-, lime-, or guacamole-flavored tortilla chips

INSTRUCTIONS:
Combine the black bean dip mix and water thoroughly. Mix in salsa and coriander. Use the tortilla chips to dip.

Mediterranean Passion Pitas

INGREDIENTS:

2 large pitas, cut into wedges

½ package instant hummus

Water as required from hummus package directions

Dash of pepper or paprika

3 tbsp. fried onion flakes

20 slices of olives

INSTRUCTIONS:

Combine the hummus mix, water, and pepper or paprika. Spread hummus on the pita wedges. Sprinkle fried onion flakes over the hummus. Top with a couple of olive slices.

Mushroom Chicken

Serves 2

INGREDIENTS:

2 ½ cups water

1 ½ cups instant rice

1 package mushroom sauce mix

1 tsp. dried tarragon

¼ tsp. paprika

8-oz. can chicken (or tuna)

1 cup dehydrated mixed vegetables (check your supermarket or camping shop, or make your own)

Salt and pepper to taste

INSTRUCTIONS:

Boil 2 ½ cups water. Remove from heat and stir in rice and dehydrated vegetables. Set aside for five minutes. Meanwhile, prepare mushroom sauce mix according to package directions. Stir in tarragon and paprika. Add chicken to rice and vegetable mixture, pour the sauce on top, and stir. Add salt and pepper to taste.

Pizza-Style Pasta

Serves 2

INGREDIENTS:

1 package tomato sauce mix (or a 14-oz. can of tomato sauce)

Water as required for sauce mix (see directions on package), plus ¼ cup if using dehydrated vegetables

2 cups elbow macaroni or other short pasta

4 oz. pepperoni, sliced

¼ medium onion, finely chopped and dehydrated (or you can use ¼ fresh onion, chopped)

1 clove garlic, chopped and dehydrated (or 1 tsp. garlic powder)

1 green pepper, finely chopped and dehydrated (or 1 fresh green pepper, chopped)

2 tsp. dried oregano

3 cups water (for boiling pasta)

(1 tbsp. oil, only if using fresh vegetables)

INSTRUCTIONS:

Prepare tomato sauce or mix according to package directions, but add ¼ cup extra water and all of the dehydrated ingredients at the beginning. If sauce is getting too thick, slowly stir in more water, one tablespoon at a time, until it loosens. Set aside and cover pot with the lid and wrap in a towel to keep warm. Boil water and add pasta. Cook for approximately eight minutes or until cooked but not mushy. Drain pasta and add to tomato sauce. Add pepperoni slices and stir.

Variations: If you have other favorite pizza toppings that you can dehydrate, you can substitute them for the onion and/or green pepper. Sun-dried tomatoes and mushrooms both work very well.

Note: If using fresh vegetables: Add onion, garlic, and green pepper (finely chopped), plus a tablespoon of oil to the pot first, and cook for two minutes, stirring frequently. Then add the sauce mix and water according to package directions, and the oregano.

Smoked Chicken Alfredo with Mushrooms

Serves 2

This is a great recipe for your first night. If the chicken is vacuum-sealed, it will last until the second night or longer in cool temperatures.

INGREDIENTS:

1 package alfredo sauce mix

Water as required for sauce mix (see package directions)

1 tsp. dried basil

1 pinch black pepper

2 cups rotini or fusilli pasta

1 smoked chicken breast (approx ½ lb.), cut into bite-sized pieces

½ cup dehydrated mushrooms (porcini if available)

1 oz. grated parmesan cheese

3 cups water for boiling pasta

INSTRUCTIONS:

Prepare the alfredo sauce according to package directions and stir in basil and black pepper. Set aside and cover pot with the lid and wrap in a towel to keep warm. Boil water and add pasta. When almost cooked, add dehydrated mushrooms for the last minute. Drain pasta and mushrooms and add to alfredo sauce. Stir in chicken breast pieces and parmesan cheese.

Beef or TVP Stroganoff

Serves 2

INGREDIENTS:

1 package stroganoff sauce mix

Water as required for sauce mix (see package directions)

2 tbsp. milk powder or sour cream mix

2 cups broad egg noodles

½ pound (before dehydrating) ground beef, cooked and dehydrated (or equivalent TVP)

½ medium onion, finely chopped and dehydrated

½ cup dehydrated mushrooms

2 oz. cooking sherry or red wine (optional)

3 cups water for boiling noodles

1 cup water for rehydrating beef or TVP

INSTRUCTIONS:

Soak dehydrated beef or TVP in cup of water for at least 30 minutes to soften. In the same pot, prepare stroganoff sauce mix according to package directions, but add ½ cup extra water and all of the dehydrated vegetables. Add the milk powder or sour cream mix, and stir in the wine or sherry as well. Simmer according to the sauce package directions. Set aside and cover pot with the lid and wrap in a towel to keep warm. Boil water and add noodles. Cook for approximately six minutes or until pasta is cooked but not mushy. Drain noodles and add to sauce.

Malaysian Satay Tofu

Serves 2

INGREDIENTS:

1 ½ cups instant rice

2 cups water

8 oz. vacuum-packed fried tofu pieces (if your supermarket doesn't carry it, try a health food shop or Asian supermarket)

¼ cup peanut butter (unsweetened is best)

3 packets of take-out soy sauce from a Chinese restaurant

1-2 packets of take-out chili sauce

½ tsp. powdered ginger

½ tsp. dried lime zest

INSTRUCTIONS:

Boil two cups water and remove from heat. Pour ½ cup into a mug or bowl and add the instant rice to the rest of the water in the pot and stir. Add the tofu to the pot but don't stir it in. Cover and let stand for five minutes. Meanwhile, combine the peanut butter with the soy sauce, chili sauce, ginger, and lime zest. Add hot water from the mug or bowl, about a tablespoon at a time, and mix thoroughly until the sauce is loose enough to easily mix through the rice. Pour the sauce over the rice and tofu and stir.

If you have extra sauce, you can keep it in a small, plastic container and spread it on crackers for snacks or lunch the next day. It will thicken as it cools.

Cheesy Chicken Quesadillas

Serves 2

These are messy but fun to eat. And they're a great escape from rice and pasta. If you're not big eaters, you can cut this recipe in half.

INGREDIENTS:

4 large tortillas

1 smoked chicken breast, cut into bite-sized pieces (or 8-oz. can of chicken)

8 oz. grated (or thinly sliced) cheddar cheese

4 oz. salsa

20 slices pickled jalapeno peppers (optional)

INSTRUCTIONS:

Heat a frying pan over a medium flame. Place a tortilla in the pan and sprinkle with ¼ of the cheese. Add ¼ of the chicken, salsa, and jalapeno peppers, and wait for the cheese to melt. Fold the tortilla in half and serve. Repeat for the other tortillas.

Vegetarian option: To add extra protein without the chicken, use some instant black bean dip or a can of refried beans.

Spiked Strawberry Shortcake

Serves 2

This is for people who prefer a dessert without chocolate. I don't understand you, but I won't judge you either! Here's a playful twist on an old classic.

INGREDIENTS:

6 ladyfinger biscuits

½ package instant vanilla pudding

Water as required for instant pudding (see package directions)

2 oz. apricot brandy

12 strawberries, fresh or dehydrated

INSTRUCTIONS:

If you are using dehydrated strawberries, soak them in hot water for five minutes to restore their plumpness. Prepare the instant pudding according to package directions in a pot or bowl. If your dishes are dirty from dinner, you can use a clean Ziploc bag to prepare the pudding instead, but be careful not to puncture the bag. Add the apricot brandy to the pudding and mix through. Arrange three ladyfinger biscuits side by side on each plate. Top the biscuits with the spiked vanilla pudding, then arrange the strawberries over the top.

Sinful Chocolate Fondue

Serves 2

INGREDIENTS:

2 bars (about 7 oz.) Toblerone or other gourmet bar chocolate

4 tbsp. cream (optional, try to get some creamers from a coffee shop)

1 oz. Triple Sec (or other liqueur)

About 20 bite-sized pieces of fruit for dipping: fresh apples or seedless oranges or dried peaches, strawberries, apricots, or pears

2 cups water

INSTRUCTIONS:

If you are using dried fruit, start by boiling up one cup of water to rehydrate the fruit for dipping. Remove the water from the heat before adding the fruit. Leave it in the water to plump up while you make the fondue.

You should melt the fondue in a double boiler, which is a smaller pot or metal bowl inside of a bigger pot. The bigger pot should have about a cup of water in it, but make sure it isn't so full that it spills over the edges when you put the smaller pot in, or so empty that it boils dry.

Break the chocolate into small pieces and then add it, the cream, and liqueur to the small pot. Place the larger pot on the burner over a low flame—as low as you can get your stove to run—then put the smaller pot into the larger pot. (Be sure to keep the water out of the chocolate, even a couple of drops can cause the chocolate to seize and ruin the whole fondue.) Stir the chocolate constantly with a wooden or plastic spoon while it melts.

Remove from the heat as soon as it is fully melted. Once you have melted the fondue, use your forks or thin sticks to spear pieces of fruit and dip them into the fondue. How sinful! Remember, if you drop your fruit into the fondue, there's a punishment. Keep some extra liqueur around and enforce the rules—drink one shot for every dropped piece of fruit!

Sex in a Pan

Serves 2

There are many recipes for Sex in a Pan, but this one is perfectly suited to camping and so satisfying it truly deserves its name.

INGREDIENTS:

8 chocolate chip cookies, crushed or broken into small pieces

2 oz. Kahlua

½ package instant chocolate pudding

Water as required for instant pudding (see package directions)

12 marshmallows, toasted (but bring a few extra, in case some go "missing")

½ cup chocolate chips

INSTRUCTIONS:

If you have a clean frying pan, you can make this in it, otherwise bring along a disposable pie plate or use a rectangular Tupperware container. Crumble the chocolate chip cookies and spread them in the bottom of the pan. Drizzle the Kahlua over the cookie bits, and mix together to moisten. Press the moist cookie crust into the bottom of the pan. Make the chocolate pudding according to the package directions, then pour it evenly over the cookie crust. Use the back of a spoon to spread it out if it doesn't pour well. Toast the marshmallows and space them evenly over the top of the pudding. (If you can't toast the marshmallows, they can be added as is or you can substitute marshmallow from a jar.) Sprinkle the chocolate chips over the top. Now grab your spoons and dig in!

Chapter 5:

How to HAVE SEX IN A TENT *Without Destroying It*

There's something about being surrounded by nature that brings out the animal side in otherwise civilized human beings. Wilderness sounds like the rustling of leaves, the breaking of waves against rocks, or even the tapping of rain on the ground, are truly the calls of the wild. At home, you can choose any kind of mood music, from Barry White to Justin Timberlake, but nothing can compete with the symphonic aphrodisiac of a thunderstorm's booming climax. Oh, baby!

It's not just the sounds of the wilderness that will seduce you. Camping has a way of making you feel more alive. The abundance of fresh air gives you a reason to take deep breaths, instead of those shallow, city breaths full of pollution. The wind in your hair and on your face makes you more self-aware. The physical challenge makes you more in tune with your body than you might normally be.

All of these things combine to make you feel more sensual and receptive than usual. Surprisingly, the harder you've been exercising during the day, the more it can stimulate your libido. After a challenging day of hiking, paddling, or climbing with your partner, you might be shocked to find you're feeling more frisky than usual. Couples therapist Esther Perel says that our accomplishments can really get those juices flowing. "Sometimes if you have just achieved something, you are emboldened," she explains. "There's a certain vitality to climbing that extra stretch or conquering a rapid. You feel mastery and joy. Mastery and joy are also what you have in great sex."

Combine that with a beautiful setting and unlimited time for privacy and intimacy with your partner, and you may never want to leave your tent. Still, there's no denying that a tent is not quite as comfortable as a bedroom when it comes to making love. Space is limited, the ceiling is kind of low, and the ground is hard and uneven. I've discovered by trial and error what I can do in there without hitting the walls, bruising my knees or elbows, or getting a very inconvenient cramp, and I'm definitely still learning. Tents may be designed to be strong, waterproof, and light, but they are definitely not made to accommodate great sex.

That doesn't mean that you shouldn't make love in a tent, it simply means that you have to give it a bit more thought than you might at home. For the majority of couples, the tent is the place they're most likely to have sex on their camping trips. (However, there are plenty of great places to have sex outside of your tent, which we'll cover in other chapters.) With a little planning and a bit of practice, you can turn the most constricting of tents into a decadent love nest, where you will enjoy some of the hottest sex you've ever had.

Setting the Mood

The buildup to a sexy night in the tent should begin much, much earlier. Whatever you are doing during the day, whether it's hiking or paddling or just lazing around the campsite, take the opportunity to add some romance. Holding hands while you walk is a simple way to let your partner know that you haven't turned into some asexual camping creature. Camping foreplay can involve anything from a simple complement to kissing and fondling. As long as you are acting like a couple, you will feel the bond of your relationship even when you have fallen silent—and that bond will turn to lust when the time is right.

If you stop for a rest or a snack, add a little hugging and kissing as well. Justine finds that some flirtation with her partner can make a big difference in her mood. "Every time we've finished a break, we have a cuddle," she says. "I usually find the going tougher than David, so he's always giving me cuddles when I get frustrated or grumpy." Hugging is far from the only option. Touching someone's hair always sends a strong signal. Or if you want to be less subtle, grab your partner's bum. Little romantic or sexual gestures throughout the day, or a bit of dirty talk if that's more your style, can get you both thinking about how you'd like to see it all play out that night.

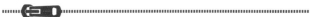

Helllooo,
Naughty Nurse!

66 One of the most romantic things a woman can do for her guy is to put something soothing on his bug bites. I'm totally serious! It's a great thing to do for anyone. We went camping in Northern Ontario once, and I guess we forgot how many mosquitoes there would be, especially since it was pouring rain. Well, my boyfriend must have been delicious to them, because they bit him mercilessly. He was just covered in bites, the poor guy. We sat in the tent and kissed while I applied anti-itch cream to each of his bites. It's a bit like playing nurse, really. And once he was less itchy, well... staying in the tent to get away from the bugs and the rain was a lot more fun. 99

—TS

How about passing the time with a playful game of I Spy? Decide on something you're bound to see now and then during the day; pick one thing each. If you're paddling, then ducks and geese are a good bet. If you're hiking, how about squirrels or trail markers? Every time you see your chosen thing, give your partner a kiss. It's way more romantic than Punch Buggy.

If you're inspired by the scenery, start to talk out a fantasy scenario. Point out places that you'd like to perform spicy acts with your partner. Is there a field of tall grass along the way where you can imagine tearing your partner's clothing off and indulging your animal instincts? Are you on a breathtaking cliff top where you could describe making love with the land dropping off right in front of you, even dangling your heads over the edge? It might be too dangerous to actually try that, but just talking about it will get you both thinking about sex. And the more you think about sex all day, the more anxious you'll be to do it when you get to the campsite—if you can wait that long!

When you're making love in the tent that night, go back to the fantasy and talk to each other as if you were actually back in those places that inspired you. Act out the fantasy, or as close as you can get to it, in the confines of the tent. You can capture some of the excitement of outdoor sexual adventures without the discomfort or the risk of getting caught.

Once you've settled into your campsite, it's time to relax and enjoy the fact that you're alone together. This is when the serious flirtations begin for a lot of couples. After a hard day of paddling or backpacking, it's hard to beat a good shoulder rub. Massage is a popular way to get in the mood at any time, but when you really need one it's just that much better. After you've had a chance to change out of your sweaty boots and socks, a foot rub might even be an option. Not only are massages sexy, they can save you from pulling a stiff, achy muscle when you're trying to make love in the tent later.

Massage can take all kinds of forms, beyond the traditional rub-down. For a titillating alternative, give your partner a flirtatious hair massage in the tent. It's gentle and sensual, and makes you more aware of how things feel against your skin. If you really don't have the long hair for it, pick a flower during the day, and lightly stroke your partner's skin with that. Start on the stomach, arms, and legs, and tease your way toward the more intimate places. Tickling the head of a penis or the clitoris with the soft petals of a flower is incredibly arousing.

The calm, quiet of the tent is an excellent place to whisper sexy secrets to each other as darkness descends. From gentle insinuations to full-on dirty talk, you can make your environment feel sexier by taking the focus of your conversation in a romantic direction. Drop the discussion about tomorrow's plans and tell your partner what you'd like to do to him or her right now. Then follow through on your promises. If you're in a crowded campground, this feels even naughtier and can help to set the mood for some sneaky, silent fooling around.

If you have trouble coming up with sexy things to say (not all of us have a way with words), bring along some reading material to help you out. Lara and her boyfriend had a long tradition of bringing books on camping trips to read out loud at night. "Most of the time we would bring a scary book, like Stephen King or something—the spookier the better!" she says. "We'd read in the tent at night, and every little sound outside would have us jumping out of our skins." They would snuggle closely after that, and the snuggling would lead to naked snuggling and more. But things got even spicier when they switched to a new genre. "A friend of mine gave me a copy of *Little Birds* by Anaïs Nin for my birthday, so I took it on our next camping trip and read some of it at night instead of a scary book," Lara says. "We could barely get through the stories without ripping each other's clothes off!"

Reading erotic stories out loud to each other makes for scintillating foreplay. Here's a hint: Women usually prefer more elaborate, romantic stories, while men tend to like more detailed sexual descriptions. Find something that turns *both* of you on. It could be anything from Anaïs Nin to Penthouse Forum. Read in your most whispery, sultry voice, or read together, each taking a different "role." It can make those long evenings at the campsite go a whole lot faster, and even if you weren't in the mood when you climbed into the tent, sexy stories might just be the thing to get you there.

Building Your Love Nest

When most people go camping, especially backpackers, they choose tents that are sturdy, weatherproof, and lightweight. Often, you don't want to carry a tent any larger than just big enough for one or maybe just a half a person. But even if you're one of those minimalist campers who like the challenge of roughing it, you might want to reconsider your accommodation when planning your love den. After all, a two-person tent isn't so heavy if there are two people to carry it. Making your tent a comfortable and welcoming space is a key part of getting

more romance into your camping trips. You don't just want to survive your trip—you want to enjoy it!

If you like to have a bit more space around you during sex, consider bringing a three-person tent. For car campers and paddlers, this won't be much of a burden, since the packed up tent won't be a lot larger than a two-person version. For backpackers, you'll have to consider the additional weight of a bigger tent. Divided between the two of you, it might not be too bad, depending on how demanding your trip is. With a larger tent, there will be more opportunity to stretch out diagonally, change positions without doing yoga, and spread your limbs a little wider. Usually larger tents are also taller, so you'll have extra head room to work with, too.

Trying to have sex in a tent of any size can seem complicated and uncomfortable at first. The ground is hard and the space is limited. You may find yourselves arguing about who gets to be on top! But there are some ways you can arrange things to be more comfortable for both of you.

Sleeping pads are important on any camping trip; they keep you separated from the cold, hard ground beneath the tent. They are also very important when you're trying to have sex—otherwise, if you're the partner on the bottom, you will feel every little rock and twig below the tent repeatedly poking into your back (and that's probably not the type of "poke" you had in mind).

Push your sleeping pads together to give you as much padded space as possible. If the pads have non-slip bottoms, this will work a lot better. Otherwise, you could find they slide out from under you on either side. Therm-a-Rest has come up with a solution to this problem. They now sell a Universal Mattress Coupler to hold two pads together. Exped sells a similar kit. Philip Torrens of Mountain Equipment Co-op explains how they work: "It's a pair of straps that hold two similarly sized Therm-a-Rests side by side to prevent rifts in the night. It will also work with other sleeping pad brands of

Honeymoon
under the Moon

For our honeymoon, my husband and I went camping at Oklahoma's Turner Falls. Although it was the week before the Fourth of July, the park was not overcrowded and we were able to find a tree-enclosed drive-up campsite.

After a fireside supper, just as the last drop of twilight evaporated from the leaves overhead, my husband came to me and kneeled in front of my chair. The kiss began softly and tenderly, and it soon gave way to a game of give and take that would lead us to lovemaking. With our lips still engaged, we removed each other's clothing, confident that we could not be seen or heard.

Even as our hungry hands played against each other's skin, the first drops of rain began to fall from the now overcast sky. Jumping to our feet, we tossed on shirts and pants and scrambled. As quickly as we could, we gathered up the firewood and food, and whatever else we could find by firelight, and stashed them in the car and tent. We dove for cover, and as we zipped the nylon door flap, the gentle sprinkling of rain escalated to a downpour.

Inside our fortress, we again shed our clothes. Our passionate embrace and the rhythm of our lovemaking were enhanced by the sound of the driving rain surrounding us. The scent of ozone and the perfect perfume of summer rain mingled with our breath in the air.

In harmony with the rainfall, and in concert with the familiar songs of the natural world, the instruments of our bodies played a tune of desire, need, and love. Our melody quickened to the crescendo of passion and softened to tender embrace. Lying there, we held each other and listened to the rain, letting our heartbeats slow. At last, we climbed between the layers of our zipped-together sleeping bags and slept.

The remaining three days of the camping trip were soggy and splendid. Our time was spent hiking and hanging out camp-side, and stealing romantic moments between storm clouds and summer sun. Eventually, we abandoned our hideaway for home. Although we could not forever stay in our rustic retreat, it will forever stay with us.

—*Donna Bowles*

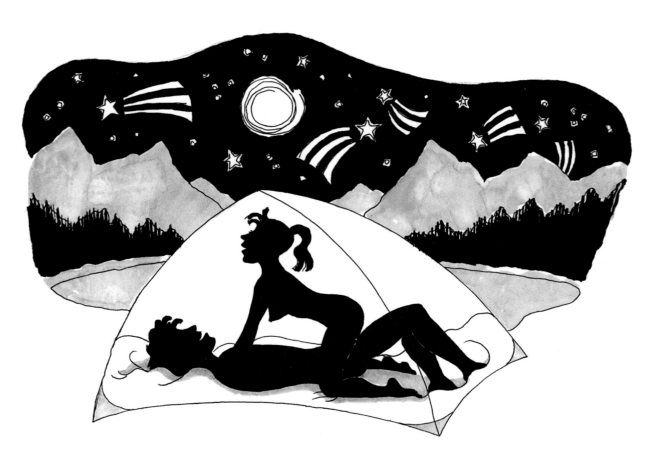

The 10 Essentials for Camping Couples

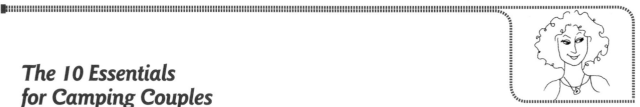

As most backpackers know, there is a standard list of "10 essentials" for camping trips. These are things you should never be without in case of an emergency, like matches and a compass, extra food and duct tape. But let's say you get stuck somewhere with your partner. Rescue is a few days away, and you've got your backpacking 10 essentials, so you're safe. Now you just have time to kill, and you want to make sure you're prepared. I have my own variation on the "essentials." Don't leave home without them!

1. WET WIPES: Whether you prefer baby wipes or moist towelettes, these little cloths are essential to give you a quick clean in the wilderness. You can get rid of the day's sweat, sunscreen, and bug spray to make yourselves more lovable and lickable, in seconds. They're also good for cleaning up after sex.

2. EMERGENCY TEA LIGHTS: Maybe you already have your all-weather matches in your safety kit. But nothing beats candles for setting a romantic mood. Small tea lights are stable and well-contained, which makes them great for camping trips. They're also small and light, so there's no reason not to bring a few along.

3. LIP BALM: Your skin can take a beating in the wilderness, and the skin on your lips is particularly delicate. Make sure you protect it with lip balm during the day, and reapply it at night so your kisses are soft and moist.

4. BREATH FRESHENER: Bad breath can really spoil the mood when you lean in for a smooch. If you absolutely don't have room for toothpaste, bring strong mints or cinnamon hearts.

5. CHOCOLATE: If you're really trying to pare down your pack weight, this can double as the "extra food" in your traditional 10 essentials kit. Chocolate helps feed your romantic appetite. Personally, I think it should be one of the basic 10 essentials for any camper, but it's even more important if you're keeping your energy up for making love.

6. LIQUEUR OR SPIRIT: It's important to make sure you're well-hydrated, so bring a water bottle *and* a flask. When you're shivering and decide to make some hot cocoa to warm up, spike it with Kahlua or peppermint schnapps for an extra dose of heat.

7. RAZOR: If you're on a longer trip, that stubble can sure get irritating. Some partners don't mind, but if your scratchy chin or rough legs are driving your lover nuts, it's nice to have the option to shave off the offending hair to eliminate the "friction" between you.

8. BIRTH CONTROL: Unless you're planning to conceive on your trip, make sure you pack some condoms or oral contraceptives. And if you're bringing condoms, don't forget the lubricant.

9. SEXY SLEEPING CLOTHES: If you stay in your sweaty daytime clothes all night, you're going to be pretty smelly after the first day—and your partner will find it hard to get in the mood. Bring something that you only wear at night, so it stays clean and dry and your partner will want to get close enough to rip it off. While you're at it, bring something sexy. Silk and lingerie are light and small!

10. "MATING" SLEEPING BAGS: If your bags zip together, you'll have a much easier time getting intimate, particularly on a cold night. It's also nice to be able to cuddle together in one bag all night, instead of separating after sex.

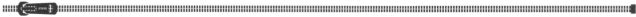

comparable dimensions. And for togetherness, ditch those weight-saving tapered pads; for proper 'docking' of pads and people, you need two rectangular pads, preferably the exact same model."

Torrens recommends buying larger pads to fill the entire floor of your tent. "It creates a bouncy-castle effect, where it's almost impossible to fall out of bed," he explains. Of course, the thicker the pads, the bouncier, so if you are car camping, or even paddling, get the thickest pads you're able to pack. Or, for a touch of luxury, look for the sleeping pads with a layer of goose down insulation, like the Exped Downmat.

If you are camping on a really cold night, you may want to keep one of your sleeping bags over the two of you to keep you warm during sex. If you buy sleeping bags that zip together, you can even stay wrapped in your pocket of warmth the whole time. Even if your bags don't "mate," you can spread one unzipped bag below you for added padding and insulation (although this will contribute to the slipping problem with your sleeping pad) and one on top for warmth. Then when you go to sleep you can each zip yourselves inside your respective bags.

The company Cocoon, which sells a variety of sleeping bags and liners that zip together to make double-sized bags, has developed a creative solution to the problem of sleeping bags slipping off their pads. They sell straps that attach their bags to sleeping pads so they don't slide around. How clever is that!

Once you've built your nest, it's time to stock it. Think of your tent as your own little honeymoon suite. With the right planning, you can create a romantic mood to beat any luxury hotel. Start with lighting. It's not necessarily a good idea to light candles in your tent, but you can create some ambiance with a carefully placed scarf or bandanna over a flashlight. If you're the type of couple who likes to see what's going on, hang a flashlight from the tent ceiling or tuck a headlamp into one of the tent pockets. (Just beware of illuminating yourselves in the tent if

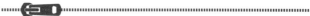

Multi-tasking with Snow Foam

66 The first time we made love in my boyfriend's new tent, he ended up with some kind of rug burn on his elbows from leaning on them in missionary position. It was pretty nasty. After that, we figured out that an extra bit of snow foam was all he needed to keep his elbows off the hard floor of the tent. Since he carries a square of it in his pack to use as a seat anyway, we just started taking it into the tent at night to use during sex. It's always nice to find a new use for something you've already packed! 99

—MG

you're camping near others—unless you're into that sort of thing.)

Be sure to keep anything that you are likely to need (condoms, lubricant, towel, etc.) where you can easily reach it. Most tents have pockets by your head, and some have a mesh shelf at the top. Leave whatever you'll be needing in one of these handy places so you don't have to start digging through bags when you'd rather be making love. Even if you prefer to make love in the dark, it's handy to have a flashlight nearby, in case you can't find what you're after by touch.

The space inside a tent is limited at best, and you're going to want to use as much of it as possible when you're making love. So avoid filling up the tent with everything you brought camping. Keep your cooking things, packs, shoes, and other gear outside the tent. If it's something that shouldn't get wet, most tents have a vestibule under the fly where you can keep your stuff relatively dry as long as the ground doesn't flood. By giving yourselves a little elbow room, you'll be much more comfy when you start getting down to business.

Before you get too distracted, try to remember to open up one of the tent windows (or vents, depending on your tent's design) to let some air in, and, more importantly, let moisture out. Just like making out in your car will steam up the windows, making out in your tent will cause condensation to get trapped inside. Your normal, overnight breathing isn't enough to be a problem, but the extra intensity of your sexual activities can leave it stuffy and even wet inside the tent if you have it shut tight. Just keep the zipper of the outer fly closed so nobody can see you.

Once things start getting hot and heavy inside the tent, there is a tendency to get focused on the fun part and not pay attention to what else you're doing. Try to be conscious of where things are ending up. Flinging articles of clothing randomly around the tent may not seem like a big deal in the heat of the moment, but it can be surprisingly difficult to find all of your bits and pieces afterward in the dark. Pick a corner of the tent for stripped-off clothing and aim in that direction. That way you won't spend as long looking for something to put on when you start to cool down after sex.

Doing the Tent Tango

While the two of you may be an orgasmic superpower in the bedroom at home, you could find that when you crawl into your outdoor bedroom, all your best moves are all wrong. What is usually hot is suddenly awkward and uncomfortable. But with a little creativity, you'll find your groove again in no time. The good news is that if you've set up your tent for comfortable sleeping, then it's also set up for lovemaking. You're on level ground, there are no big rocks or roots in your back, and you're sheltered from the wind. So how are you going to have great sex without knocking out the pegs or tipping the whole tent over? No problem! Just keep to the center and try to remember where you are.

In terms of position, your options will be somewhat influenced by the type of tent you're in. If your tent is a very low, tunnel style, you'll have to keep a low profile yourselves. Missionary position works well, as does a lying down, woman on top. Just be careful in missionary; the woman will have to keep her feet on the ground or wrapped around her partner. If she spreads her legs wide, she's likely to press against the walls of the tent. That could cause damage to the tent in the long run, and on a rainy night it could also cause a sudden indoor flood! If the woman prefers to be on top, give this a try: She should lie with her chest against her partner's and drag her hips upward toward his navel, then come back down with a circular motion. This will give her maximum clitoral contact and make it easier to reach orgasm if your tent is too low to sit up and get deep penetration. Oh yeah, and it's pretty good for the guy, too!

If head space is very limited, sometimes the most comfortable position is spooning, with both people on their sides, man behind woman. This is also one of the best positions for keeping warm, since you can both stay under a sleeping bag and share body warmth without the risk of a draft. In this position, it's easy for a man to reach around his partner and fondle her breasts or use his fingers to give her extra pleasure on her clitoris. So what it lacks in eye contact it makes up for in other areas. Spooning is the easiest method for two men to use in this kind of tent as well. Again, you've got the option of an easy reach-around. Even two women can make this position work for them, although they might prefer to lie face to face on their sides. Feel free to throw one leg over your partner for better access, but beware of hitting the side of the tent.

As Priya points out, the spooning position is also the easiest for keeping quiet in a busy campground. "Spooning makes the least noise when trying for all we're worth not to make it obvious!" she says. "To be crass, bite hard if you're a screamer." There's not much you can do to help a screamer, unless she's OK with a ball gag or you don't mind getting bite marks. Your best option is to make love as far as possible from other campers.

Once you've found a good position and the two of you are going at it, try to shift your weight or slightly change your position now and then. Staying in the same position for too long may cause your legs, hips, or back to cramp up—not quite the muscle spasm you were hoping for! By adjusting yourselves every few minutes, your muscles should stay looser and everything will go a whole lot smoother.

If you're the kind of nature lover who likes to "bush-whack," or "lollygag," as the case may be, you may find oral sex a bit challenging in a confined space. Most tents are not much longer than one body length, so if one of you tries to slide on down, you're going to hit the foot of the tent. The simplest way around this is the classic 69 position, with your feet at opposite ends of the tent (although you'll have to at least unzip the sleeping bags, or one of you is going to find it very stuffy). If you have a reasonably tall tent, a woman can kneel, straddling her partner's head, while he performs oral sex on her. Unfortunately, this position doesn't work as well for men, although it can be done. It becomes more of a modified 69 in that case, with him facing his partner's feet and putting his hands down on the floor of the tent.

Another position to try for fellatio in a tallish tent is kneeling beside your partner's head. Or, if neither of you is very tall, simply find the longest diagonal line along the floor of the tent and have your partner straddle your legs and bend over you. That can work for cunnilingus as well, but with the man (or other woman) kneeling between her spread legs rather than straddling.

If all of that seems a little too complicated, you can keep foreplay simple by going for manual stimulation instead. You can always just snuggle up in your sleeping bags, or under them, and fondle each other to your heart's content.

However you decide to make love, don't leave out the afterplay. It's a bit of a letdown if you've just had great sex and then you zip yourselves into separate bags. If you've got a double bag, cuddling is no problem. Otherwise, try to leave the top half of your bag unzipped, so you can still reach over and touch each other. If you sleep really close to your partner, the open bags won't get too chilly. If you absolutely need to zip up for warmth, you can still play footsies through your bag. It's not quite as intimate, but it's still letting your partner know you're there.

While nighttime is the easiest time to go unnoticed by other campers, some couples prefer to have morning sex on a camping trip. They feel more confident and attractive in the morning because they haven't had a chance to get dirty and sweaty yet. Not to mention that on very active trips, they're just too exhausted at the end of the day. If you've gone to sleep at sundown, you'll probably be waking up very early anyway. It never hurts to put the time to good use. Making love in the morning also has the advantage of a bit of daylight in the tent. You'll have an easier time finding what you need, and cleaning up after yourselves.

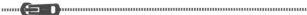

Top 10 Euphemisms for Making Love in a Tent

1. Answering the *other* call of nature

2. Painting the canvas

3. Howling at the moon

4. Keeping the bunnies awake

5. Working off the marshmallows

6. Driving in the tent pegs

7. Sharing body heat for survival

8. Gathering wood

9. Shakin' the stakes

10. Flapping the fly

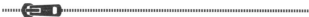

Tentus *Interruptus*

" There are some dangers when you borrow a tent from friends and you aren't used to it yet. So let this serve as a warning to everyone—make sure you try putting up the tent at least once before you go out camping with it.

We started getting busy in the tent after a long day of hiking, and things were pretty passionate. My husband was on top and we were kissing like mad. There wasn't a lot of space in the tent, I have to say, and when he tried to roll us over so that I was on top, he rolled us onto the side of the tent. I guess we didn't do a very good job of putting it together, because somehow one of the poles popped out of its place! The end of the pole must not have been sitting properly in its little grommet. It was already getting dark when we set up our campsite, so we kind of rushed, and, as I said, it was a borrowed tent we'd never set up before.

The next thing I knew, I was on top of my husband, naked, and the tent was caving in on us. He didn't want to stop, but I was laughing too hard to keep going. I mean, how can you have sex when you're literally wearing your tent? At least there was no damage to the tent. I couldn't imagine trying to explain what happened when we returned it to our friends. **"**

—*OB*

Keeping It Clean

There are also things to consider as far as sexual hygiene goes. Some campers use condoms when they're in the tent, just to avoid mopping up afterwards. Don't like sex with condoms? Maybe it's time you tried it again. If you've been out of the condom market for a while, you might be surprised by the range of options.

Stephanie is a condom convert. She's on the pill, so normally she doesn't use condoms with her husband. But to keep things less messy, they use condoms when they're camping. "We make it a bit of an experimental thing," she says. "If we're going camping, we try to find some interesting kind of condom we haven't tried before and see what it's like—ribbed, flavored, or whatever! It's become sort of a camping ritual to go into a sex shop and find something really outrageous we've never seen before. If there's no new kind of condom on the shelf, then we'll go for a new lube instead."

If you're not sure where to begin, don't be afraid to ask for some expert advice. I asked Nicola Mercer, the director of d.vice designer sex gear, what she would recommend for a camping trip. "I would buy an assorted pack, and that way you can try a whole bunch of different types, and you're trying something new and making it a bit of an adventure," she says. She suggests some of the options to look for. "There are different sizes and different sensitivities–ultra-thin, which increases sensitivity, which is what most men complain about. Different textures, different flavors—it makes it fun for both people," she adds. Along with getting the right type of condom, Mercer emphasizes the necessity of lubrication. "People often don't think to use lubricant with a condom, and that's why they don't enjoy them," she explains.

Condoms do make it easier to clean up after sex, so why not give them another try? You may be surprised by the results. Pack out your used condoms in a sealed plastic bag, with your other garbage. Never dump them down the outhouse hole or bury them.

Keeping a barrier between you and your sleeping bags and/or pads is also a good idea. "Try laying a large towel across the crucial hip area of (your sleeping) pads before you lay anything (or anyone) else," suggests Philip Torrens of MEC. "That way you can both bathe in the afterglow rather than the aftergoo." Torrens recommends using a quick-drying micro-fiber travel towel rather than a cotton one. "It can be washed and drip-dried off the

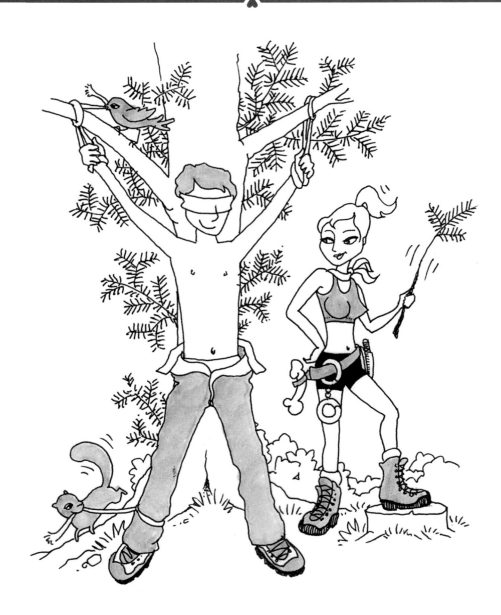

Not Even
Sweet

❝ I think of two things as the English bird gives me a blow job inside my dome tent. One: How much noise are we making? We got Security Dave in the tent to the left of us, and Long Lost Larry, with his kids, in the tent to our right. The last thing I need right now is the whole surf camp listening to the English bird moaning like someone from an Austin Powers movie.

The second thing I'm thinking about is Christine. Where is she right now? What is she doing? Is she at it with another guy back in Montana? Is she thinking about me at all?

"I find you terribly sexy," the bird whispers.

"Um, thanks." I never know how to respond to her breathy compliments.

There's an hour difference between San Diego and Missoula. Chris is probably still at work. She's serving last call, preparing to clean up.

The bird takes her mouth off my business for a second and coos, "You drive me absolutely mad!" I think she means crazy. She doesn't seem mad.

Now, there are several reasons why I haven't had an orgasm in three months. Some sort of misguided fidelity to Christine kept me from pursuing any of the female clients who have come through the camp this summer. The reason I haven't been servicing myself is a bit more complicated. It has to do with a story that Security Dave told me about his first year working at surf camp. He said that the second time he went to pleasure himself, he reached for his cleanup towel and almost instantly felt a tingling sensation all over his body. When he turned on his lantern, he found that the rag was infested with thousands of tiny ants.

"More ants on that rag than on any candy wrapper or soda can I've ever seen around here," Security Dave told me.

"They like that stuff?" I asked. "It's not even sweet."

"Protein, Dude," Security Dave replied. "It's protein."

After the ants had their fill of the rag, they proceeded to march in formation over to the source of their food—the innocent nether regions of Security Dave.

I don't know how true this is, but every time this summer that I have even considered taking myself out for a date, I feel a crawling sensation all over my skin and immediately think better of it.

So you see, after almost the entire summer of deprivation, my member is a loaded gun, a loose cannon in the hands of a skilled English bird who is showing no mercy. Yes, indeed, the bird knows what she is doing. She's no slouch.

"Oh, baby, does that feel good, Darling?"

I am tempted to answer her truthfully: No. It just eases the pain. But I think better of it. I close my eyes and try to concentrate on the forthcoming orgasm.

The bird's all hands now. Faster and harder, moaning as though she's the one about to come.

"Oh!" I don't know if she says this or I do. I'm too focused on the moment of release. My whole body tenses.

"Oh, yes, Darling..." Three months of self-denial erupt, splattering the bird and reaching the roof of my tent. An obscene amount of semen leaves my body. I would be embarrassed if I weren't so relieved.

For a moment, I wonder what the bird thinks of me now. Not darling. Not beautiful. Not sexy. Just an ordinary guy who really needed to blow his load. Certainly nothing to put up on a pedestal.

Then she breaks my thoughts. "Sweetie?" the bird seems disturbed. "Do you feel something crawling in the mattress?"

"Ants," I reply, though I'm not really bothered by them.

"A...a...ants?" She tenses up. "What are they doing?"

"They're coming to eat the protein."

"Protein?"

"That's right. Protein."

"But it's not sweet."

"No, it's not sweet. In fact, it probably tastes bitter. But they need it to survive. It's life."

I think this philosophical line of reasoning might impress her. But the bird screams and runs out of the tent, presumably toward the bathroom. She manages to grab a towel on her way out.

I stay on my mattress and feel the little scavengers crawling all over me, eating my seed. They are in a feeding frenzy, and I am the most relaxed I have been all summer. **99**

—*Tyler McMahon is an editor of Surfing's Greatest Misadventures (Casagrande Press).*

thwart of your canoe or the back of your pack during the day, ready for repeat rutting by nightfall," he says.

Wet Ones or baby wipes are also handy to have around for cleaning yourselves up after sex, or anytime. If you do end up with a wet spot on your sleeping bag, blot it with a damp towel (or some absorbent clothing or tissues) right away so that the moisture doesn't seep into the filling. That goes for both body fluids and excess lubricant. You can do a better job of removing any residue from the surface of your bag later, but you don't want it to have time to soak into the loft, or it'll have to wash the whole bag when you get home. Sleeping pads are more resilient, and depending on the kind you choose, you may not need to worry about damaging them. "Closed-cell foam sleeping pads are wipe-and-go as far as post-passion puddles are concerned," says Torrens. Fabric-covered pads are more likely to absorb some liquid, so try to wipe them off right away.

Toys and Tools

A lot of couples use sex toys and other extras as a regular part of their home sex life. It can be a challenge to safely incorporate these things into a camping trip, and a bit of a pain to bring a large amount of regalia along with you. Traveling light is important for camping, after all. But that doesn't mean you have to abandon all of your favorite sexual practices when you leave home.

The first thing to do is prioritize. Which pieces of sex gear will you miss the most if you don't bring them along? Consider size and weight, particularly if you are backpacking. Perhaps one dildo will do instead of your whole collection. If the trip is a short one, just a night or two, it may not be worth the bother of bringing toys along at all.

For those who want to pack something small, Nicola Mercer of d.vice designer sex gear suggests a silicone cock ring with a mini-vibrator that fits into it. "The vibrating (rings) are great for couples because they vibrate against the guy who's wearing it and whoever he's having intercourse with," she says. "So they're a great couple toy. They also tend to have a removable bullet (vibrator), so in terms of value for your packing money, if you're going off into the mountains, you take a small bullet with a cock ring it fits into."

The other main consideration is cleanliness. It's hard to keep things clean in the wilderness, and when it comes to dildos, vibrators, or anything you're planning to use for any kind of penetration, you've got to make sure you can keep it clean enough to avoid giving you or your partner a nasty infection. The easiest way around this with dildos and vibrators is to bring condoms and place a fresh one over the dildo every time you use it. That way, you never come in contact with the surface of the dildo, and don't even have to worry about cleaning it afterwards.

If you choose to use toys without a condom, clean them with soap and warm water, then give them another rinse to get rid of the soap residue, and dry them with a towel. If you're worried about the cleanliness of the water available to you, boil the water first, then let it cool a bit before using it. Make sure your toys are completely dry after cleaning to prevent mold growing, and then store them in a sealed plastic bag. Keep them in your pack well away from things like cooking fuel and bug spray—anything you wouldn't want to apply to your insides!

If you use a dildo or buttplug (or anything else) for anal penetration, I strongly recommend using condoms, particularly if you are going to use it on both partners, or use it vaginally as well. Technically, you could kill any bacteria by boiling the dildo, but who the heck wants to go camping with an extra pot just to keep their sex toys clean?

If you're into dildos but don't want to pack a lot of extra stuff with you, consider using biodegradable alternatives. A carefully selected carrot, zucchini, or cucumber can make a great sexual aid. Just cover it up with a condom when you're using it, then the next day it can be part of your lunch or dinner. You don't even have to pack it out with you!

Vibrators can be a lot of fun, although you may find that they detract from that "back to nature" mood out in the woods. The first thing that you're likely to notice is that the gentle buzzing noise that seems so innocuous at home, sounds much louder in the silence of the outdoors. "When you're in the store (choosing a vibrator), you can compare that sort of stuff," says Mercer. "The reality is that even the quiet ones, on a quiet, still night, if anyone's near you they are gonna hear it."

So make sure that there isn't anyone else around, say within 50 yards of your tent, if you're going to be using a vibrator. If you know you won't be alone, maybe it's time to think about silicone instead. If you thought dildos were just for gay couples, think again. Mercer was surprised by the sales patterns in her sex toy shops. "The majority of dildos we sell are to heterosexual couples—around 80 to 90 percent," she reports. Why? They allow straight men to experience penetration, they give monogamous women the chance to feel different sizes inside of them, and they also take the pressure off in terms of men getting an erection on demand.

If you're trying to keep things small and light but don't want to be without a vibrator, consider bringing a fingertip vibrator instead of a dildo-style one. It will take up less space and be lighter to carry. While it can't perform all of the same functions as a dildo-style vibrator, lots of women rate them highly for nipple and clitoral stimulation and they can be held against the testicles or perineum for added effect during fellatio. You can also try a "bullet" vibrator, which is a small, cylindrical shape, or a vibrating cock ring.

Inevitably, bits of dirt will make it into your tent as you go in and out, so never put your sex toy down on the floor of the tent. If you do, it will need cleaning before you use it. And don't forget to lubricate! Lube should be applied any time you use a toy for penetration, to avoid irritating your skin. An internal infection is unpleasant at the best of times, but if you're several days away from medical attention, it's going to be torture. As with dildos, the

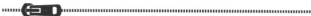

If a Vibrator Buzzes in the Forest, **Will Anybody Hear?**

" We have a few sex toys at home. We both enjoy using them on each other, and they really add to our lovemaking. So if we go on vacation we always bring at least one toy along, just for fun. After all, that's when we really have the time to enjoy sex!

One of the first times we went camping together, we brought our bullet vibrator, since it's nice and small. It's also waterproof, so we could wash it up easily. We thought we were pretty clever, actually!

Our campsite was pretty close to our neighbors, but we figured we'd just wait until they went to sleep. About an hour after the tents on either side went dark, we got all cuddly and started making love. My wife pulled out our vibrator and turned it on. It was so loud, it woke up the neighbors. I'm not kidding!

The light came on in the tent next to ours and I could hear them asking what the fuck was that noise? I started giggling as she quickly turned it off and we sat in our dark tent, hearts racing, until they'd settled back down again. We ended up putting it away for the rest of the trip, and next time we brought a nice, quiet ostrich feather instead. **"**

—TD

easiest solution to protecting yourself from infections is to cover the vibrator with a fresh condom and lube each time you use it. Then as long as you're far away from other campers, and you've got a supply of batteries with you, go nuts!

Another small toy that's easy to pack is a cock ring. These are good for keeping the guy's penis harder, longer. They can be as simple as a leather or rubber strap, or come in a variety of silicone shapes and sizes. There are even models that have a built-in clitoris stimulator, so every time the man thrusts, a little piece of silicone tickles his partner's clit. How thoughtful! And don't forget the vibrating models that give an extra thrill to both partners.

Lubricant is not technically a toy, but it's something to keep in mind when you go on a camping trip planning to have sex. If you're going somewhere or traveling at a time when you expect the conditions to be particularly dry, like on a desert or a winter trip, you might find lube handy, even if you don't usually use it. For anyone using condoms or sex toys, especially if anal sex is in the picture, it's pretty much a necessity. Lubricants can be either water- or silicone-based. Traditionally, the silicone-based ones have been more popular for anal sex since they're a little more viscous. But a good water-based lube is easy to clean up, effective, and shouldn't leave you feeling sticky until your next shower. Like anything with a high water content, very cold temperatures could make it freeze up, so keep it well-insulated in your pack if you're doing any winter camping.

If you've forgotten your lube, don't try to improvise by using other products like Vaseline or sunscreen. They can damage your condoms or possibly you. The next best thing if you don't have lube is lots and lots of saliva. Mercer also warns against buying some of the more gimmicky lubricants on the market—after all, you're putting this stuff in your most sensitive places. "If it's got sugar in it, keep away from it; if it's flavored, keep away from it," she says. The chemicals added to these novelty lubes can cause unexpected reactions. So if you're keen to try one out, give it a test run well before your camping trip. That way you'll know whether you are likely to have a reaction to it. "A lot of people have nasty responses to (novelty) lubricants, even the warming ones," says Mercer.

When you are using lubricant, be careful not to spill it all over your tent. Keep the lid in your hand while you are using the bottle, so that you don't drop or misplace it in the tent. You don't want to put the festivities on hold while you search around for a tiny, plastic lid. You should

Romantic Camping
Gift Ideas

Is your partner's birthday coming up? Or Christmas, Valentine's Day, your anniversary, or any of the many, many occasions that seem to require buying a gift? It can be hard to think of fresh ideas after a while, so here are some things your co-camper might enjoy receiving from you:

DOUBLE SILK SLEEPING-BAG LINER: This will give your nights in the woods together that luxurious touch of class. You might just feel like the couple on page 123, and enjoy it so much that you start to sleep in it at home, too!

LEXAN WINE GLASSES: If you like to drink wine on your camping trips, these lovely goblets will turn every dinner into an "occasion." They're not for the hard-core light packer, but if you don't mind the space they take up, they sure look a lot nicer than a coffee mug.

BLINDFOLD: Everyone has enough room in their pack for one of these—even you lightweight types. A blindfold is helpful when you've been up late (having sex in the tent, of course) and don't want to be woken by the first rays of the sun. And they're also lots of fun for sexual play!

HAMMOCK: If your partner doesn't have a lightweight hammock yet, it makes a great addition to your camping kit. Be sure to get a double size so you can use it together. They're great for lazing around the campsite, or flip to page 132 for some sexy ideas to get you into the swing of things.

CAMERA: Digital cameras come in all shapes and sizes these days. Having one that fits into a pocket makes it easy to bring and use on camping trips. Now your partner can capture all of those beautiful places you're visiting together.

Plus, you can get involved in some "candid" photography at the campsite if you're feeling playful!

CAMP SHOWER: Having a shower in the backcountry is luxury, indeed! Not only will your partner feel better after a good rinse, but you'll be able to reap the benefits by getting close and cuddly without having any nasty odors to deal with.

NATIONAL PARKS PASS: Depending on where you live, there are various passes available to allow you access to parks on an unlimited basis. Having annual passes gives you one less thing to think about when you're planning your trips, and if you're camping together regularly, you'll definitely get your money's worth.

LINGERIE: If you're the woman, buy a slinky nightie or teddy to slip on in the tent, and your man will probably think it's the best gift he's ever received! If you're the man, buy something silky for your lady and tell her how much you'd like to see her in it on your next night in the wilderness.

GUIDEBOOKS: This may not seem like a romantic gift at first, but explain that it will give you the opportunity to discover the destinations of your dreams, and your partner will probably catch on. Buy guides for places you really want to visit together, even if it's somewhere you'll have to save up for. Appendices 1 and 2 may give you some inspiration to begin with.

ROMANTIC COUPONS: If you're strapped for cash, or your partner has literally everything, try making some personalized coupons for your lover to use. They can entitle him or her to free kisses, shoulder rubs, foot massages, oral sex, or whatever you're willing to redeem!

look for a lube with a flip-up cap, or try transferring your lube to a small travel bottle with a flip-up cap, so you can avoid taking the lid off completely. Just make sure you label your bottles if you are taking things out of their original packaging. You don't want to confuse your lube with the dish soap.

For couples into BDSM, you may find things a bit limiting inside your tent. There is nowhere to tie anything to that won't result in bringing down your tent. Simple toys like handcuffs and blindfolds are easy enough to use in the wilderness, but more extravagant games may have to be left at home. Mercer suggests basic wrist restraints. "Generally, having hands above the head and bound together gives a good feeling of bondage," she says. "Or you could get a branch and attach your restraints to each end of that with string, and you could have more of a splayed-wrist bondage."

If you bring along a few well-chosen ties or scarves, you'll have a ready supply to use for blindfolding and restraining. Other items that you can pack along in small spaces include nipple clamps and thumb cuffs. If you're a careful packer, you might even be able to take along an ostrich feather or two.

If you feel the strong desire to satisfy a foot fetish, and traditional camping footwear is just not doing it for you, be wary of the stilettos. There's a reason you never find high-heeled hiking boots on the market. They can easily tear a hole in your tent, including the floor, with very

little force, or even rip through your backpack. Be equally cautious with riding crops, whips, paddles, and other things that tend to get waved around. There's not a lot of room for error, and the consequences can leave you cold and wet. But then again, if you're into pain, this might just heighten the experience for you. It may be best to find a secluded spot outside the tent for anything that requires swinging room.

Remember that with BDSM, most of the fun is in the atmosphere and your attitude, and you can create that yourselves without a lot of props. Use tone of voice to change the dynamic of power and restraint. But have a discussion about what you want to do first. You don't need to have a box of toys if you use your imagination.

Any couple with a passion for the outdoors and a sense of adventure will find plenty of ways to indulge their desires while they're out in the wilderness. These suggestions should get you started if you are uninitiated, but soon enough you'll be finding your own special techniques.

We'll get into more sexy activities in the following chapters that can all happen *outside* the tent. The possibilities are almost endless when you leave "polite society" behind. The most important things are to talk to your partner about what is a turn-on for him or her, and to be considerate of the other campers out there. If you keep your eyes and your minds open, you'll never run out of opportunities for great sex in the great outdoors.

Chapter 6:

Making Car Camping the ULTIMATE DRIVE-IN

Last year, I hurt my foot and couldn't do a lot of walking, just as summer was beginning and all I wanted to do was go camping. Backpacking was out of the question, and even a paddling trip had to be put off because it was too hard to climb in and out of a boat. So the only thing on the calendar for several weeks was car camping.

It had been a while since I'd done any car camping, and both Gerhard and I realized on our first trip of the summer that we'd forgotten how comfortable it is. You can bring great stuff like lawn chairs and cold drinks, not to mention bottles of wine, fluffy pillows, and other romantic aids. The only drawback was that it got more challenging to find a place where we could get a little privacy. It seemed like everyone and their dog was out there with us. So we started driving all the way through the campgrounds to find the most private site. Then we'd pitch our tent in the corner farthest from where anyone in the neighboring sites might pitch theirs.

As it turned out, car camping was a lot better than I remembered it. One of the nicest things about it is that you can bring along all of the luxury items that are too heavy or bulky for backpacking or paddling. Some of these things can definitely help make your camping experience more romantic.

Luxury on Four Wheels

Car camping is an occasion for indulgence. When you're bringing your car, there's no reason to skimp, since you've got lots of space and won't need to carry anything. This is your opportunity to build your own luxury resort.

Start with the tent. While backpackers and paddlers will usually take a small, two-person tent to save space, you've got the option of stretching out. Consider bringing a three-person (or even larger) tent to give you extra elbow room. Larger "family" tents are also taller, so you will be able to move around inside more easily. Some are 6 feet or higher. Many large tents come with a covered vestibule area, where you can sit outside

while it's raining and still stay dry. These are great for cooking under, too.

Even if you're used to a tight squeeze, you might find, as Jessica did, that it's much more comfortable to supersize your tent. "The first time my husband and I shared a tent, it was a one-man and we were squeezed in tight and cozy," Jessica says. "We were young and uninhibited and only wanted to have a good time. Now we have a huge family tent and a lovely air mattress with a battery-powered pump." If you're looking for a spacious tent, check out the offerings from companies like Eureka and Wenzel, which have lines for people who like a little wiggle room.

Next, make sure you have a cushy bed. Even the thickest of backpacking sleeping pads can't compare to an air bed (although Therm-a-Rest is now making a luxury pad that's 2.5 inches thick.) It's the difference between a Swedish mattress and an Army cot. A nice, thick mattress can make you forget about the hard ground below when you start getting down to business.

If your tent is big enough, you can even have a queen-sized bed to stretch out on. Before you faint from blowing all that hot air, take some comfort in the fact that a lot of models now come with built-in pumps so that these lofty beds self-inflate. (You'll want to save your "blowing" energy for more fun activities.) As for getting you off the ground, Aerobed makes a model that's 19 inches high. If you and your partner are finicky about your cushioning, look for models with separate valves for each side so that one person can sleep on a softer mattress while the other has a firmer one.

You also don't need to settle for simple sleeping bags when you car camp. Priya and her husband get decadent with the sleeping arrangements on their outings. "We bring along a duvet instead of sleeping bags, and with a blow-up double mattress and fluffy pillows, there you go!" she exclaims. Now all they need is room service.

For author Kathleen Meyer, bedding down with her man just isn't romantic if she has to use a lightweight sleeping

Romancing the Campground

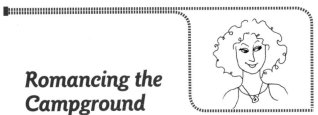

If you think that the caravans packed with wailing kids and whirring generators make romance next to impossible at a campground, you're missing out on some great opportunities. When I was stuck with a hurt foot and nowhere to go but the "family" campground, I figured out some great ways to turn those trips into romantic escapes:

– Play on the swings at the playground at night, after the kids are all in bed.

– Lie on the hood of your car together staring up at the stars. If you see a shooting star, don't forget to kiss and make a wish.

– Kiss with a piece of ice from the cooler in your mouth.

– Walk around the campground after dark and make up erotic stories about the people in the tents.

– If it's raining, go for a walk anyway. Wear your sandals so you can jump in the puddles.

– Sneak into the showers at night and have a close encounter of the hot, wet kind.

– Come back to your tent in the middle of the day (while everyone else is away doing daytime activities) and make love.

– Rent a canoe and pretend it's a gondola. Serenade your lover with cheesy, romantic songs. Bonus points if you sing in Italian!

– If the campground laundry doesn't close, make love late at night with the woman sitting on top of the dryer while it's running.

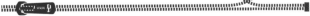

bag. "I find it really hard to deal with nylon-lined sleeping bags," Meyer says. "It's not inspiring to be romantic in that at all. I like flannel sleeping bags because I think it's cozy." Since Meyer and her partner spend most of their nights outside, even at home, comfort is important. The tall couple have extra-long bags that they zip together, so they can cuddle in their comfy, flannel pocket.

Seating options open up for car campers, too. Packing a couple of those canvas, folding chairs can allow you to spend a whole evening by the campfire without once losing the feeling in your bum. Double-chairs are now available for that cozy "couch" effect. And if you prefer to snuggle, you can pick up an inflatable loveseat to elevate your comfort level. Just make sure it's one that's designed to be outdoors, or a puncture could put an end to your cuddling.

One of the nicest luxuries on a car camping trip is a hot shower. For campgrounds without shower facilities, you can either buy a camp shower (see Chapter 3), or bring along a portable water heater that runs off a propane tank. These compact devices have a spray nozzle to make showering easy. Suddenly car camping seems awfully civilized, doesn't it? You can even bring a portable chemical toilet. No more excuses about having to stay at the most developed campgrounds. Now you can take your own facilities with you and get away from those crowds—and you won't need an RV to do it.

You can bring the feeling of luxury to your outdoor meals as well. Most drive-in sites have a picnic table. Bring along a plastic tablecloth, or even a large towel, to make the switch from eating to "dining." Lexan wine and margarita glasses are available at a number of camping shops, so you can add a touch of class to your outdoor cocktails. Mountain Equipment Co-op and REI even carry a manual blender made by GSI, so you can make icy drinks like daiquiris at your campsite.

Coffee makers are available in all shapes and sizes for campers, so if you're picky about your java, you're in luck. Espresso makers and basic percolators for campers have been around for a while, and there's even a filter-style coffee maker that works just like the ones people have at home. Lexan coffee presses are also a good pick for those who don't like to percolate. They're available in a full range of sizes and styles. Cowboy coffee full of grounds is off the menu these days.

Avoiding the Family Free-for-All

The couples I spoke with while writing this book consistently told me that their most romantic trips were the ones with the fewest other people around. They described trips where "we had the whole place to ourselves," "it was completely deserted," and "it felt very private and romantic." Obviously, being alone leaves you with a lot more options for expressing your romantic side, but what if you can't ditch the crowd?

Trying to get away from it all is great, but when convoys of people try to get away to the same place at the same time, you've got to put in a little more effort to keep things romantic. As I see it, even if there are a hundred people all around you admiring the starry sky, it doesn't mean you're going to see fewer stars than if there were just two of you. You just have to block out everything except for your partner and enjoy where you are.

Usually, this works just fine, but my good friend, Tobey found ignoring the neighbors quite a challenge on her last trip with her husband. "On a wide-open field, the sound from the other campsites carries really far," she grumbles. Even though they picked a spot far from the other campers, they were annoyed by the music blaring from a group of teens across the field. And just when they thought it couldn't get any worse, the group was joined late at night by two more friends arriving on roaring motorcycles. Luckily, the noisy group moved out in the morning, but morning seemed to arrive way too early that day. "Earplugs come in handy," Tobey advises.

Many campgrounds are laid out with trees strategically planted to keep the noise from echoing around the sites.

If you find yourself camping on a flat, open area, expect to hear the neighbors. On the bright side, if they're noisy and blaring music, they won't be able to hear anything you get up to in your tent!

For a romantic car camping getaway, you'll want to be where the crowds aren't, if at all possible. That means doing your homework ahead of time to find the ideal location. With a little planning, you can grab yourselves a secluded corner and hide away so you can feel like the only people around.

A few things can almost guarantee a big crowd at the campground. Accessibility is a big one. If a nice camping spot is within half a day's drive from a major city, it's going to be crowded every weekend over the summer. The easiest way to avoid these crowds is to make a little extra effort. Go somewhere a bit farther away, where most people can't be bothered going with their three kids in the car making them crazy. While it may take you longer to reach your campsite, the time you spend there will be so much more peaceful and intimate, you'll be glad you went the extra distance.

Sometimes the longer drive can seem to take forever. Instead of feeling like you've wasted a day, try to leave early in the morning and break up the trip. Stop at a park or forest along the way and take a romantic hike together. If you can time it right, pack your lunch and find a quiet place to enjoy a picnic. And if there's nobody around, you can sneak in a little "afternoon delight." Then you can return to your car refreshed and ready to carry on to your final destination.

Another way to find some peace and quiet is to stay at an "adults only" campground. These places cater to couples, from honeymooners to retirees, in search of childless solitude. They may not have as wide a range of facilities, like swimming pools for instance, but they will have an abundance of silence.

Chris McCallum, owner of the Wild Duck Campground in Scarborough, Maine, believes that couples enjoy the environment at his campground because it gives them a chance to quietly appreciate each other's company. "In the stresses of daily life, that can easily get lost or misplaced with the constant interruption of the telephone, or outside sources of stimulation such as the TV or the needs of children," says McCallum. "It's nice to rekindle that flame or rediscover the reason they are together and why they fell in love."

To maintain this sense of solitude, Wild Duck has a separate area for tent campers, so they aren't overwhelmed by huge RVs with growling generators. "They have their choice of a shaded, secluded site, or we have an open grassy area if they prefer the sun," McCallum explains. "And when they want to just sit by their campfire and enjoy a quiet conversation, there is not any hustle and bustle around them at any time during the day to prevent that."

While family campgrounds often encourage interaction among guests with community centers and playgrounds, adult-only campgrounds are happy to let their visitors keep to themselves. McCallum has learned to give his guests their space. "I greet them with a smile when they arrive, and a friendly wave during their stay, but grant them their privacy because they are here for them not for me," he says.

Even family campgrounds can offer some solitude if you choose well. Ask around and see which places have separate tent camping areas. Some family campgrounds even have an adult section away from the families. Ask whether their layout keeps each of the sites separated or if you'll just be in a big, open field. Find out if they are on a quiet river or lake that doesn't allow motorized watercraft like jet skis, which can spoil the feeling of tranquility.

Ask about the details of the individual campsites as well. Will you have a fire ring? A picnic table? Can you get a site on the waterfront? The more you ask for specifics, the better the odds that you'll get what you're after.

Private Parking in Public Parks

Some large wilderness areas have been turned into national or state parks in order to protect them for future generations. Most of these enormous parks have more than one campground, and usually the campgrounds closest to the park entrances fill up first. Booking ahead might be necessary in the top parks, and in some places every available spot can fill up in high season. But in larger parks, sometimes there are more remote camping areas hidden away from the main entrances. Find out if there are less-busy options, and don't be afraid to ask park staff where the most private campsites are. You may have to stay somewhere with fewer facilities available, but the tradeoff can be a camping trip spent in quiet seclusion.

In fact, some parks have car camping sites with no facilities at all apart from an outhouse. The French like to call it *camping sauvage*. (It always sounds so sexy in French!) To most of us, it's "primitive camping." It's a great compromise between the comforts of car camping and the privacy of backcountry camping.

If there are no alternatives, ask the park staff to assign you to a campsite in the farthest corner of the campground. Stay well away from high-traffic areas like playgrounds, laundry facilities, and shower buildings. If the campground isn't full, you may find that hiding in a remote corner actually gives you a lot of privacy.

Some parks are so popular that there is just no way to find any privacy on summer weekends. If you're determined to visit one of these places, try planning your visit off-season. By avoiding summer, you'll often find you have the place to yourself. Parks take on a whole new life in the autumn months, when the trees show their glorious fall colors, so think about packing an extra fleece and waiting for the crowds to disappear. If you're not too fussy about maintenance, early spring can also be a good time to visit popular parks. In fact, you're likely to see the parks in their most "natural" state before all of the summer preparations begin. On the down side, this could mean dealing with fallen trees across the road, mudslides, and other obstacles that have appeared over the winter. So if you're going on an early spring trip, take your sense of adventure with you.

One factor that brings in the crowds is a natural icon. If you make plans to see Old Faithful at Yellowstone on a summer weekend, you certainly can't expect to be alone. The places that everyone talks about are bound to be the busiest. So if it was in last month's *National Geographic*, forget it. If you're looking for some privacy, seek out the less-publicized spots, where the busloads of tourists won't be stopping for their fifth photo opportunity of the day. Regardless of where you live, there will be plenty of places to explore, but people tend to gather around a small number of specific sites. That leaves a whole lot of less-crowded areas for you and your partner to enjoy.

If you're dying to see those iconic places, you can stop and see them for a couple of hours, then get back in your car and drive to a more isolated location to make camp for the night. As long as the sights are on or near a road, there's no reason why you have to spend the night right beside them. You can also visit those places during the off-season. Just call the park ranger and find out when is the least-crowded time to visit.

It's much easier to plan a car camping trip away from the crowds if you don't have your heart set on any particular park. Ignore the glossy brochures and take a good look at a map. Where are the hidden gems, the little parks that nobody knows about? Join some online forums where campers discuss their favorite spots. (There are websites with forums listed in Appendix 3.) Ask the staff at local camping shops and outfitters for advice on "secret" places to camp. You may have to sacrifice having a hot shower, but you will probably find beautiful areas of wilderness you never even knew were there.

Luck can also play a part in finding the campsite of your dreams. When Gwen and her husband took a long weekend trip, their reserved campsite was in a crowded state park. But along the way, they got hopelessly lost. "We'd been driving for something like five hours, and we really should have been there already," she says. "I wanted to turn around, but then my husband saw a little camping icon that pointed us down a side road."

But they were not heading toward the state park. They were actually getting farther and farther away. "The sign actually led to some wilderness area we'd never even heard of," recalls Gwen. "We stopped the car, and had a look around. It was on a gorgeous lake, and there was practically no one there, even though it was a long weekend. So we found a campsite there and had one of our best camping weekends ever!" They've been back to their secret campground many times since then, but they refused to tell me where it is, because they're afraid if it shows up in a book it will get too crowded.

If you own a four-wheel-drive vehicle (I know there are a lot of you out there), even more choices are open to you. It's time to finally get some mud on that SUV! There are roads and trails you can take that are not an option for the minivan crowd. In fact, some campsites accessible by four-wheel-drive tracks are as isolated as backpacking sites. There won't be any facilities, but there won't be any other campers, either.

If there's a four-wheel-drive club in your area, find out where the off-road trails are, and if any give you access to campsites. You can also check in local bookstores and camping shops for guides to the area. There may be specialized maps, and in some cases entire books, that will show you where the off-road trails are and what sights lie along the way. Going off the main roads is a sure way to get away from the crowds, and if you've already invested in a vehicle that can handle it, you might as well use it.

Campground Sexual Etiquette

If, despite your best efforts, you end up with neighbors at your campsite, it doesn't mean you have to abandon the idea of having sex (nor do you have to invite them to

Sleeping
in the Sage

She thought I was never coming back. In Seattle, we slept late with the windows fogged and the damp creeping in under the doors. We took walks in the mist and rain in this place where gardens bloomed all year long. We swore without ever making a promise that we were together. But we knew that nothing was ever going to happen here. We both loved the sun. It was too much for me, the rain, the idea of being so much in love I was about to let go, to give up the defenses, and let her in.

Then I left for the desert. I dried out in the sage. She didn't believe that I wanted to be with her, and I knew it. How could I convince her? Say it? Anyone can do that. Instead, I studied the high desert and wrote back to her so that it could be hers, too.

I told her how rabbit brush bloomed like yellow fire in the dry, cool spring. How you can hear the burst of meadowlark song when you drive along the fence lines at 80 miles per hour with all the windows down. Told her that thousands of years ago people lived along the Snake River plains who saw the earth split open and folds of lava bleed out. That they left rock circles and flakes of obsidian that were still secrets here. Told her that if you crushed sage between your fingers it smelled clear. That it wiped away all that rain and the heaviness of our Seattle lives. Told her how sage grouse puff up their necks and dance in circles and you can pull up at night and turn off the lights and watch them.

I told her that the sagebrush had different names: *Artemisia tridentata*, three-toothed Big Basin sage;

Artemisia wyomingensis, short, twiggy, low sage that hid songbird nests and wasp eggs. Those names were mythical: Artemis, the huntress, goddesses of the moon whose dogs would rip to shreds any man who saw her naked skin. Tridentata, the trident, three-tined symbol of Poseidon, whose vast ocean had once stretched out even here and left fossils as its testament in the rock. Told her, too, that there are canyons here, deep and unclaimed, that drop from nowhere in the middle of nothing. Told her that after it rained here, everything woke up.

The more I looked at that cold sage desert, the more I found in it. I swear I fell in love more seeing the desert for her, filling her with it. And I did come back, and told her that I had to bring her here, to this place I had learned to love through her.

So we drove through the traffic and the heavy pull of the cities of the coast. We drove over the Cascades, out of the clouds. It was night when we hit the desert, but we kept driving, until we could barely stay awake. By the time we set up our tent, it was cold and felt almost like a dream. We slept together in it with the windows open so we could feel the night breeze and see all the stars. And in the morning, we woke to a meadowlark and we smelled like sage and the desert was all around us. And it was ours.

—Doug Schnitzspahn is a writer and editor living in Boulder, Colorado, with his wife, Radha (to whom he proposed on a camping trip while scaling 14ers in the Sangre de Cristos), and two children.

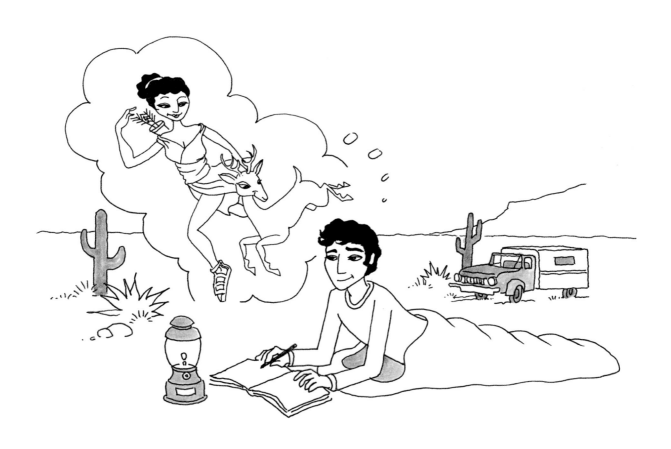

A Little
Morning Glory

66 We went on a camping trip with some friends over the July 4th holiday. It was a lot of fun, and we stayed up late telling stupid jokes around the campfire and drinking beers. The only problem was my boyfriend and I were totally in the mood to have sex, but we had our friends in the tent right next to ours. I just couldn't deal with them listening to us, and I knew I'd never be able to stay awake waiting for them to fall asleep. It was a real drag.

But in the morning when we were all still in our tents, we decided to go for it. As far as we could tell, everyone else was still asleep. We kept as quiet as possible because we knew our friends were just a few feet away, and we thought we were doing a pretty good job of it.

While we were right in the middle of having sex, someone woke up and got out to go to the washroom. When she got back, she asked if we were playing footsies in there because our tent was moving. Later on, she admitted to me that she knew exactly what we were doing in there! **99**

—DA

join you). On the other hand, basic campground etiquette suggests that you do not start screaming, "Give it to me baby!" at the top of your lungs. People go camping to find a little peace and quiet, so be respectful of your neighbors.

The first thing to do if you are in a busy campground is find an isolated corner for your tent. If your neighbors have already put up a tent, try to pitch yours as far from theirs as possible. You shouldn't sacrifice basics like level ground for this, but do the best you can. If there's nobody next to you yet, but there is clearly another campsite beside yours, try pitching your tent as far away from the neighboring site as you can. Have a look at the next site to see if there is an obvious place for people to pitch their tent. Most people will go for the flattest, clearest spot. If you have a fair idea of where their tent might go, you can figure out the best place to pitch yours for privacy. If you get lucky, nobody will end up using the site, but it's better to be prepared for someone to show up, since moving your tent later on would be a pain.

Once you've got some privacy, campground sex is all about keeping a low profile. If you usually require music to put you in the mood at home, you may need to rely on the more subtle sounds of nature when you're camping. Music carries a long way through a quiet campground. This is doubly true late at night after most people have retired to their tents. While it's tempting to rely on music to drown out any other noises coming from your tent, it's considered bad form to force other campers to listen to your tunes.

If you absolutely need music to make love to, bring a small, portable source such as an MP3 player with speakers. Put it right next to you in the tent and keep the volume down. If you're not sure how low the volume needs to be, turn the music on and then walk to the edge of your campsite, where it connects with the nearest neighbors. If you can still hear it, you need to turn it down.

Campfires are one of the most romantic parts of a night in the woods together. Snuggling up in the glow of your fire is a lovely way to pass the evening. If your campsite is reasonably sheltered, you can even get a bit more intimate in front of the fire. But it has to be said that stripping off your clothes anywhere that you are visible to other campers is a no-no. Campfires provide a significant amount of light in an otherwise unlit area, so if you're fooling around by the fire, anyone passing by will have their eyes drawn in your direction because your fire will be the brightest thing around. Back out of the glow completely before you start to take off any clothes, or simply throw a blanket over you and be discreet.

If you've decided to retire to your tent to fool around but are worried that your quivering tent may attract the attention of your neighbors, stick to positions like spooning that don't require large movements. If it's warm enough, push your sleeping bags to the side or foot of the tent so they won't rustle beneath you. And remember that if you turn on a flashlight inside your tent, your silhouettes will be visible. So unless you want everyone to see what you're up to, turn out the lights.

You might also find that light sources outside of your tent can be distracting when you're trying to make love. When other campers walk by with their flashlights on (or under the light posts that are installed at some campgrounds), they may appear much closer to your tent than they really are. You could see the shadow of a passer-by falling across the wall of your tent, and wonder what kind of pervert is lurking right outside watching you. The reality is that shadows from low light sources, like flashlights, can stretch a long way. That person you think is standing right outside your tent is probably 10 feet away or more. Once you've got yourselves tucked inside the tent and turned out the lights, you're ready to flip back to Chapter 5 and try out a few of the suggestions.

To be supremely subtle with your copulation, some women find that just by squeezing their pelvic floor (pubococcygeal or PC) muscles with an upward motion, they can create an internal thrust. This means that once he's penetrated his partner, the man doesn't have to move at all to get friction against his penis. You may find that this technique requires a bit of practice. It doesn't work for everyone, but it's the most silent and secretive way to have sex. (Not only is it good for camping, it's also great if you're stuck in a guest room with a squeaky bed!)

Women can work their PC muscles using Kegel exercises. The exercises are simple. Just squeeze inwards and upwards, like you're trying to stop yourself from peeing after you've started. Do 10 squeezes, five times per day. You can do them at your desk, while you drive, or while

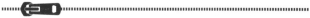

Revenge of the Trucker Kitty

66 My boyfriend was moving to Calgary from Toronto, so we packed all of his stuff into his pickup truck, grabbed his cat, and went off to camp our way across the country. On our first night, we stayed at a little campground just off the highway and we made love inside our tent.

When we were done, my boyfriend suddenly sat upright and said, "Why is it light outside?" We'd been so engrossed in each other, we didn't notice until after, but it was light out. He popped his head out of the tent and realized that his truck headlights were on.

Somehow the cat, which we'd left inside the truck for the night, had managed to pull the lever by the steering wheel and turn on the lights! From then on, the cat stayed with us in the tent overnight. **99**

—AM

you're watching TV. Or if you're not the exercising type, pick up a set of Ben Wa balls or love balls (described in Chapter 3), and just keep them inside your vagina for 10 minutes to half an hour a day for a couple of weeks.

If you are big on the idea of making love outside at your campsite, wait until complete darkness has fallen. Find the most sheltered area of your site, behind some trees or between your tent and some trees. While one of you sits in the place you've chosen, have the other person wander out to the common pathway or road (check for well-worn shortcuts as well) and see if you are visible to others. If not, you're safe to get naked there, as long as you get back inside your tent before dawn breaks.

Picnic tables are a favorite spot for sex among adventurous campers. If your table is too visible, this might not be an option, unless you can do it in the cloak of darkness.

Just clean up the dinner plates and you're free to make an extra meal of each other! The best thing about making love on a picnic table is that you're outside but not lying on the cold (possibly rocky) ground. Throw a sleeping pad on top of the table, and it's an instant outdoor bed. What could be hotter than making love surrounded by nature with the stars shining down on you?

If you both get right on top of the table, you can use just about any sexual position you like. Either partner can be on top, or you may even fit side by side. Another good position to try is one I like to call "Setting the Table." Have the man stand and the woman lie down with her hips at the table's edge. She can lie either face up or face down. For a variation of this, the woman can also stand and bend over the table with her partner entering from behind ("Clearing the Table" position).

Of course, picnic tables are designed so you can sit and eat, so why not use them for oral sex, too? One partner can sit on the edge of the table, feet on the bench, while the other partner, the giver, faces the receiver sitting on the bench. It works for everyone, and it's one of the most comfortable positions for oral sex you're likely to find in the wilderness.

Your car is another good place to have sex, if you park it far enough onto your site. It's not as private as your tent, thanks to all of the windows (that is, until you steam them up), but if it's dark enough outside, you should be able to have a tumble in the back seat unseen. It's like being a teenager all over again! You can relive those nights of fooling around, away from your parents' prying eyes. You'll also have the bonus of being able to turn on your car radio for music, since the closed doors will keep the sound inside.

You may want to leave the windows open a crack, so they don't fog up and give you away, but of course that will make you easier to hear. So you have a choice between keeping quiet with good ventilation, or being louder and steamy.

The key to having sex at your campsite, in or out of the tent, is to keep it to yourselves. Try to avoid really loud vocalizations, or thumping against anything that makes noise. And as I mentioned in the last chapter, vibrators are louder than you might think. The rest of the campground is going to be very quiet at night, so any noises will seem louder than usual.

If you know that you and your partner are loud when you make love, then only do it where there are not other campers around. This may mean going farther off the beaten track than you're used to. If you're really big on having loud sex in the wild (and who can blame you, it's fun!), consider taking up backpacking or paddling so you can reach more isolated campsites.

If you're more adventurous with your sex life and would rather not worry about what other people think, you may want to consider a more specialized camping trip or campground. There are all kinds of clubs and groups around the country that hold their own sexually open camping trips—trips where having sex in public is all part of the fun. It may be just the answer to your exhibitionist dreams!

There are usually separate events for straight and gay campers, with the gay events generally for either lesbians or gays, although some groups offer "mixed events." The group will book out a large area, usually a whole campground, so that they can make their own rules and not worry about what is acceptable to the general public.

You can find very specific practices at a lot of these events. Some cater to swingers and group sex, while others specialize in BDSM. Some specialized campgrounds are open to nudity, and some to sexual freedom, all of the time. Again, these vary from exclusive places for gay men, or lesbians, or just anyone who wants to walk around naked.

If you are very open with your sex life, this could be just the thing for you. You'll have to do some research to seek out these places and events in your area, but you may

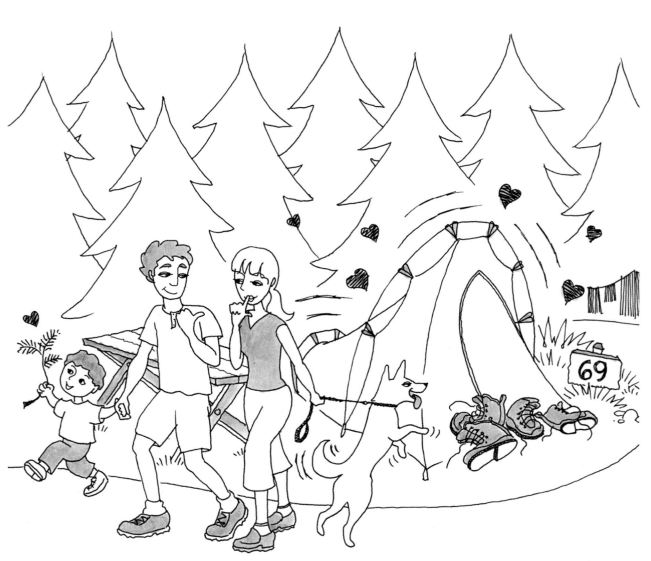

be surprised by how many there are. Gay outdoors clubs are a good place to start if you are looking for same-sex events or locations (but remember that not all gay outdoors clubs are about hooking up for sex), and if you are straight, you can find details through swingers clubs or BDSM groups.

If you decide to join one of these outings, check out the rules first. Every group has its own set of rules and etiquette to make sure that people can enjoy themselves with no uncomfortable surprises. No matter where you are, or what group you're with, no means no. If you make people at an event feel pressured or uncomfortable, you'll probably be asked to leave. On the other hand, don't go to an event where you will be uncomfortable. If you aren't into BDSM, it's a bad idea to join a group trip where that's the theme just because you're looking for a place where nudity is allowed. Also, talk to your partner about it ahead of time and choose the group or location that's the right match for *both* of you.

Going Out of Bounds

If you're in a busy campground but you don't like the idea of having sex near the other campers, it may be better to seek out a more private spot to be together. Wander away from your campsite and look for other places nearby where you can be alone.

At state or national parks, there are probably some hiking trails that start from or near your campground. Taking a secluded trail is a good way to put some distance between you and the crowds around your campsite. Unfortunately, even hiking trails can get busy during high season, but the farther you get from the main campground, the thinner the crowds will be. Speak with a ranger about which trails are the least crowded, or check the park map and find a trail that is longer and more difficult—a surefire way to avoid others. Make a day of it and pack a lunch.

You may find yourself reaching new heights, like Heather and her husband, who achieved more than one climax

atop Arizona's Table Top summit one day. "Though we were not the only ones hiking the Table Top Summit Trail that day, we were the first ones to reach the summit, at 10:20 that morning, after hiking for two hours," she recalls. Figuring that the other hikers were at least a half an hour behind them, Heather and her husband sought a secluded area away from the sign post, stripped down to nothing but their hiking boots and sunglasses, and got busy. "We were dressed long before the other hikers reached the top," Heather says. "By that time, we were eating lunch and admiring the scenery." Not bad for a morning's walk in the woods.

Unless you plan to make an early start, it's best to drive farther into the park to find less-traveled trails. If you're in a park with a network of roads, the trails starting at road ends well away from campgrounds will have the fewest people. Even if you've put some distance between you and the nearest tent site, you may still run into other hikers, so getting naked right along the trail is a risky proposition. Try going off-trail a bit to find some more privacy. Tall grass and thick forest can provide enough cover for the two of you to fool around or have sex unseen. We'll get to more detailed ideas for off-trail romps in Chapter 8.

You'll also have better luck on trails that are not marked as dayhikes, but are the starting points of longer, multi-day routes. Just remember to turn back in plenty of time to return to your campsite before dark—unless, of course, sneaking away in the dark was your plan all along. If you've got flashlights and a good sense of direction, wandering away from the campground at night can give you the privacy you're after.

Val has her own favorite way to take a nighttime stroll: "What is especially nice, is walking in the moonshine in the middle of a road that runs through a forest—naked, of course, and holding hands."

A few parents also admitted to me that they sometimes waited until the kids were asleep in the tent, then snuck away for a tumble on the beach, or behind the bushes.

My friend Sam and her boyfriend find opportunities for lovin' in the camp facilities. "My boyfriend and I are way more adventurous when we're out camping," she says. "I think all of that fresh air must go to our heads! Our favorite place to make love is by the campfire, but we can't always do it if there are other campers around. So usually that's just for paddling trips."

Their favorite place for sex while car camping? In the shower. "We'll wait until most of the campers have gone to bed and sneak off to the showers," Sam says. "If they're empty, we'll go in and have a romp. If we're feeling really naughty, we'll do some role-playing, too, and pretend it's a school dorm or something. I've snuck him into the girls' dorm, and we're hiding in the bathroom so we can have hot sex! It's always kind of exciting because you can't be sure if someone will walk in while you're making love."

If the shower's not your thing, but you like the idea of water, you could bring or rent a canoe and use it to find your own private spot in a park. If you are on a lake or river system, paddling away from the main campground opens up the whole park to you. Instead of being limited to a marked trail, you can pull up to shore anywhere that seems tempting and enjoy the scenery however you want. Bring a ground sheet and some soft stuff, like jackets, fleeces, or life jackets. Suddenly, you've got a nice, comfy place to have sex or just enjoy the solitude!

Regardless of where you go, car camping will give you ample opportunities to experiment with new places to make love. It will also give you and your partner the chance to indulge and pamper each other with luxuries you can't usually take on backcountry trips. But romance and seduction are all about your state of mind. As long as you're both feeling sexy, you'll have no trouble making it work for you.

Chapter 7:

Paddling to
PARADISE

Canadian historian Pierre Burton once famously defined a Canadian as "someone who knows how to make love in a canoe." At least two of the couples I surveyed from north of the border claimed that, yes, they have done the deed in a canoe. And as someone who was born and raised in Canada, I hope to someday master that art myself. As it stands, I can't even get a canoe to go in the right direction! At the risk of having my passport revoked, I admit to having failed (so far) at this most Canadian of activities. But enjoying some romance on the water (or next to the water, or in the water) is easy, even if you don't have the agility and balance of a Cirque du Soleil acrobat, or the strength and power of a Wayne Gretzky slapshot.

Fortunately, you don't have to be Canadian to be a great paddler (or a great lover). And once you start, you'll realize that paddling is one of the best ways to get away from it all. It's also the ideal transportation for two.

There are a lot of advantages to camping this way as a couple. It's much easier to find a private, isolated campsite along the water's edge than by sticking to the roads and trails. Just think of all of those paddle-in island sites! It's also an easier way to transport your gear than backpacking, so it opens up the world of backcountry camping to people who might not have the strength (or the desire) to carry everything they need on their backs.

There's something inherently romantic about paddling—the quiet of your surroundings, and the graceful motion of the canoe or kayak. It's like being in another world, somewhere between earth, sky, and water. You have a unique opportunity to appreciate the stillness of nature. In this frantic age, nothing is more romantic than sharing that tranquility with your partner.

How to be Romantic When You're Not Even Facing Each Other

If you're paddling, particularly in a two-person kayak or canoe, it can feel like you're barely interacting with your partner. You're not facing each other and not touching for most of the day. How the heck are you supposed to be romantic when you're staring at the back of your partner's head for hours on end? No problem! All it takes is a bit of imagination.

Since you can't look at each other, you'll lose some of your natural shyness, which will allow for different ways of communicating—like flirty or dirty talk. Bait your lover with a titillating list of things you'd like to do when you get to solid ground: "I want to lick the saltwater off your body. Bury you in sand and then give you a strip tease. Roll with you on the shore as the waves lap against our naked bodies."

Paddling is a great time to let fantasy take over. Lose yourself and be inspired by your surroundings. For me, paddling on calm waters makes me think of a 19th century setting where lovers in rowboats sneak away from their high-society garden parties. Where are they going? What are they going to do? Have they abandoned their turn-of-the-century morals to indulge their secret passions? Top hats are tossed aside and more than a little ankle will be revealed.

If repressed passions and frilly hats aren't your thing, try pretending to be a knight or a gypsy, rescuing your royal lover from a horrible, arranged marriage. Whatever your fantasies, this is a great time to share them with your partner. There's no pressure to act on them right away, because you're busy paddling. But if you can both get into it, a good erotic fantasy can turn into an elaborate story over the day, and leave you both ready for action at night.

You can add to the sexual tension by reaching over and touching each other once in a while. Dip your hand in the water and gently caress your partner's breast or leg, or simply lock eyes now and then. But don't go too far. Your goal right now is to build up desire and anticipation of what's to come.

Couples therapist Esther Perel says the anticipation of fantasies can be as much of a turn-on as sex itself. The build-up gives you plenty of time to get hot and bothered. "You can imagine things the way you see them happening later," she says. "Anticipation is that kind of forethought. The fact is that in nature you can't always control things, and you have to finish one thing before you can do some-

thing you want. You have to get to a certain spot in the river before you can stop. You have to set up the camp." Perel believes that a little fantasy-based sexual tension can make things feel more erotic between two people. "Eroticism is sexuality transformed by imagination," she says. "The essential ingredient is imagination."

If you prefer more structured fantasies, here's another game you can play while you paddle. You've heard of Cinderella's fairy godmother? Become your partner's fairy godlover! Grant him or her three wishes, to be fulfilled later that evening. Or maybe they're wishes that could be fulfilled the next time you get out of the canoe for a break—or even in the canoe. Stuck for wishes? Here are some suggestions: A 10-minute foot massage. Making love that night without breaking eye contact. Having your hair brushed. Being fed trail mix while resting your head in your partner's lap. Oral sex by the campfire. Making love completely naked, even if it's cold in the tent. Got some ideas of your own? Excellent, now you just have to decide who gets to wish and who gets to grant wishes. (Just a hint, it's nice to take turns.)

If you're the kind of couple who don't like to beat around the bush, skip the role playing and just talk about things you'd like to do to each other later on. It doesn't have to be sex talk all of the time. Even planning to light a campfire and have a glass of wine later can keep you romantically connected during the day.

Wet and Wild

During a summer paddling trip, you can't beat going for a swim together as a way to reconnect. It's both playful and sexy to glide through the water together and splash each other. Or take turns chasing each other, and when you finally catch your partner, the water will hide you if you want to touch each other or strip your suits away.

If you have time, pull the canoe or kayak up on a beach and strip down to your bathing suit (or your birthday suit). You'll finally get a good look at your partner after

Role-Playing Games for Water and Beach

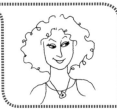

There's something about water that is universally erotic. It's fluid and free. It makes us feel uninhibited and playful. For me, water invites fantasy. Depending on whether I'm paddling down a river, gliding naked in a swimming hole, or chasing my lover through the waves, I might engage in one of these games to suit my mood.

Mermaid temptress and a sailor

Persuade the pirate to reveal his hidden treasure

Victorian lady and her handsome stable boy row away for a tryst

Convince the cannibal to let you live

Summer camp runaways with a stolen canoe

Adventurers exploring the Nile, or the Amazon, or the Mekong

Survivors drifting in a lifeboat

Voyageurs ready for business at the trading post: What do you need? What will you trade?

Naughty stowaway

Shipwrecked virgins of the Blue Lagoon

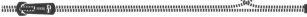

hours of staring at the back of his or her head. Take a long look before you head for the water. You've probably been having sex in a pitch-black tent. When was the last time you got to see your partner's body in sunlight? Go ahead and admire! It will make both of you feel more attractive.

Once you're in the water, you can just splash around, or you can fool around. It's up to you and how long you've set aside for your swim. Even a quick dip can involve a bit of kissing and caressing. You'll be feeling cleaner and smelling better, so why not take advantage of it? Of course, if you have time, you can take things much further.

If you're into wet adventures, make sure you veer away from heavily used areas. If you're traveling along a river, or along a hiking trail that runs parallel to a river, chances are others will wander by. Try to find a sheltered spot or a less-used area. If you are camped near water, wait until dark and go for a nighttime swim to make love. The starry sky will heighten the mood, and even if there are other campers on the same lake or river, they won't be able to see what you're up to. Just remember that sound can carry farther on water because there's nothing to block it, so keep your voices down if you want to remain discreet.

Before you dive in, a word of caution about sex in the water: Some medical professionals discourage people from having sex with their privates submerged because the man's thrusting can force water into the woman's uterus. This can cause serious infections, particularly if the water contains dangerous bacteria or viruses. While most people don't seem to have any problems, it's important to take the risks into account before you take the plunge.

If you've decided to go for it, there's the question of how to have sex without drowning yourselves. (And for you non-swimmers, it might be best to try sex in the bath before graduating to deeper waters.) Sex in the water can be a balancing act, especially if there are waves crashing around you, or if there's a strong current.

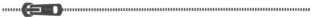

A Nice Day for a Wet Wedding

66 My wife and I actually met through our love of paddling. We were introduced by a friend of hers whom I was working with. I was talking with my colleague at lunchtime one day, and I told her I was going on a canoe trip that weekend. She said, "Oh, you should meet my roommate— she's been canoeing since she was a baby."

Well, it turned out we actually had a lot in common (unlike a lot of people I've been set up with), and of course, paddling has always been part of our relationship. We got married four years ago, and we had the ceremony in Algonquin Park in Canada. Everyone had to canoe in, so we got these big voyageur canoes and all paddled to the wedding site in our formal wear. It was fantastic! My grandmother seemed a little mystified, but everyone had a great time, and frankly, any other kind of wedding just wouldn't have been "us." 99

—RE

One of the most stable positions is for the man to kneel in shallow water (shallow enough for his shoulders to stay above the surface) and the woman to wrap her legs around his waist and hold onto his shoulders. Or the woman could squat over him with her feet on the bottom. Doggie style can also work in shallow water, and has lots of stability points so you can deal with breaking waves around you. If there's no water movement, try it with the woman more upright, in the reverse cowgirl position rather than on all fours.

If you're stable enough to stay on your feet, you can venture into deeper water. You'll want to be about shoulder deep, or a little shallower if there are big waves. Nothing spoils the mood like getting smacked in the face by a breaker! The woman can again wrap her

Holding the
Ace of Hearts

We were four women in our 30s and 40s, and we'd come to Baja on our annual girls' surf trip in search of surf, sun, and release from endless emails, Evites, cell phones, and complications of life in San Francisco. We came for yoga on the beach after a day of surfing, and for the ritual filling of our bellies with fish tacos. We came to revel in the outdoors and forget the disappointment of the online dating scene and divorce, and maybe, just maybe, we'd find a little romance.

As it happened, we had landed in a campsite of vagabond surfers who drifted in from Australia, Italy, and Vancouver Island to ride the giant swell that had come in for the week. The camp was occupied by mostly men in their early 20s who were traveling from swell to swell in broken-down vans. They strutted around, shirts off and surf shorts riding low to reveal exquisitely sculpted muscles. Each day, my friends and I took turns surfing, and in between breaks talked about the "taco de ojos" (eye candy).

Then one night, I met my match—the Boy. Sitting before me, headlamp pushed jauntily to the side of his forehead, tousled bangs covered with sand, he focused intently on the playing cards fanned out in front of him. He had invited himself into our group, and now this decidedly younger man was teaching us how to play Hearts.

But there was something about being in Mexico that made me think that maybe he could. At home, I rarely initiate matters of the heart, but this time it felt different. I had spent the week harnessing a different kind of power, working all my muscles to drive my board again and again into the

break, fighting a strong current, twisting and turning in the foam until I finally surfaced to that sweet sucking of air that comes after being held under.

I felt powerful and sexy, and my senses came alive. I could taste the spicy burn of the taco hot sauce. I could feel the heat radiating off my skin from days in the sun wearing next to nothing. There was something about the taste and smell of salt on skin and hair, something about watching beautiful bodies curve their surfboards into the green liquid. There was something about the magic of letting the night and the beer do the final work of relaxation and romance.

As we ended our last hand of Hearts, just three of us remained. Annelie yawned loudly and said she was going to bed. Then the Boy stood up and stretched his arms skyward. "You gonna go to bed, too?" he asked, casually raising an eyebrow. This was the crucial moment, and I could feel it, like a riptide, starting to float away. Before I could answer, I saw two streaks of light shoot over his shoulder. I gasped. "Did you see that? Those shooting stars?"

The next thing I knew, we were laying on a thin blanket outside his tent, avoiding cacti spines and spiders. I nestled myself into the crock of his arm, and we both shivered as the desert night turned chilly. We took turns identifying the obligatory Orion and Seven Sisters and continuous shooting stars in the infinite blue. I felt the heat of our bodies begin to fuse. His lips softly brushed mine and came to a stop, slightly parted. I tasted salt and tequila. As our lips locked, our bodies moved closer, and the weight of his long, bony

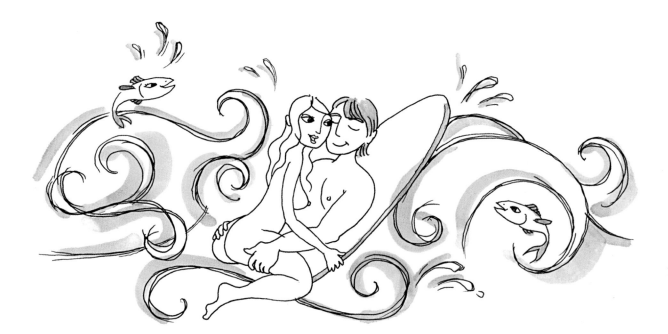

joints were almost painful as they rested on my neck and thighs. Warmth and tenderness from his kisses flowed through the length of my body.

I could feel his heart pounding through his chest. "Can you hear the waves?" he asked, pushing my salty hair away from my face. I strained to hear the crash of the 20-foot swell the storm had ushered in. "Yeah," I whispered, as our bodies rocked to some unspoken rhythm. With eyes closed, one ear on his chest and one to waves, I was suddenly back on my board, feeling the waking of water beneath, waiting for the next wave to break. I smiled to myself. Finally, this was one hand of Hearts that I was not going to lose.

—*Meg Moser is a nurse, backcountry skier, and surfer in San Francisco.*

legs around the man's waist, and since the water provides buoyancy, she won't seem to weigh a thing. Or, if you are similar in height, she can keep one foot on the bottom and her partner can lift the other leg up around his hip.

Before you start to mess around, make sure you can bail yourselves out if you get interrupted by a nosy bystander or curious sea life. Priya learned the hard way that water play is best left for private moments. In a trip with her extended family, Priya and her husband were shoulder deep in the water getting ready to get it on when, she says, "My granny, of all people, came waltzing over." The pair could just barely hide the fact that they were stark naked. But something in their faces (horror, perhaps?) told Granny these weren't the most welcoming waters, and she turned around. I bet Granny was no fool! She probably had her share of naked swims back in the day.

Getting naked is the easy part, but some sexual acts require more creativity. Oral sex can be challenging in the water since we can't keep our faces submerged for long periods of time. It's that silly need to breathe that ruins your fun! The easiest way around this is for the receiving partner to stand in shallow enough water to expose his or

Marriage Breaker vs. Honeymoon Maker

Canoes and kayaks may seem like the perfect way to travel as a couple, but they have also earned the nickname of "marriage breakers." At first, paddling with your partner is a bit like making love for the first time. You're only going to succeed if you manage to get into a matching rhythm and forge ahead at the same pace. Failing to find your groove together will leave you both feeling frustrated and disappointed. If you're new to canoeing or kayaking, or to sharing your boat, you may need to get back to basics before you end up in a battle of the paddles.

Choosing the right boat is the first step toward paddling harmoniously. A tandem kayak is the most dependent on teamwork because you are seated close enough for your paddles to clash if you are not in synch. Therein lies the power struggle, as the person in front sets the pace, while the person in back has to follow (so deciding who gets the front is a bit like deciding who gets to be on top). If you have major differences in your strokes, seek out a kayak with the cockpits farther apart to minimize the clashes until you even out your cadence.

In a canoe you are usually far enough apart to avoid physical conflict, but since the stern paddler gets to steer, that can be a source of contention. Make sure the stronger, more experienced paddler takes up the rear position. If you're both keen paddlers, play nice and take turns. And remember, nobody likes a front-seat driver!

If you just can't seem to get it together in the same boat, think about taking solo canoes or kayaks. That way you can each pick your pace and control your own direction. And believe it or not, being in separate boats can make it easier to have a conversation. Pulling up beside your partner to chat is much more effective than twisting around in the canoe, or shouting up to the front. In fact, a lot of paddlers' shouting matches start out with the two people just trying to hear each other.

Making the right choices before you hit the water can make the difference between romance and relaxation, and a battle of wills. You'll need to have some patience and a sense of humor on your first few trips together, until you find your rhythm. After that, it's all floating downstream!

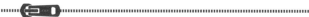

Up the Creek
Without Any Clothes

❝ Around noon, we found the mother lode of all campsites, set in a cave (so it was well-sheltered and very secluded), about a hundred feet from the creek. We had lunch, then we went skinny-dipping in the creek. While splashing around in the water, we were suddenly aware that people were approaching on a nearby trail.

We hid behind boulders and watched as a whole group of backpackers passed us by—there were seven of them, one of which was an elderly woman. Not all of them saw us, but the ones who did, including the elderly woman, only smiled and waved. We did the same, because what else are you going to do in such a situation?

Instead of getting out of the water and putting our clothes back on, we stayed where we were and continued to skinny-dip. *Again* we were caught as the last of the backpackers passed us by. They only whistled at us then continued down the trail. ❞

—Heather Verley

her genitals. The giving partner can then kneel in front, or squat, and it's pretty much like doing it on land.

For a different experience, you can try having the receiving partner lie on his or her back, floating in the water. Some people are better floaters than others (generally women float better due to our distribution of body fat), so the giving partner may have to help out by supporting the receiver under the thighs or bum. This position gives you the chance to experience a whole new sensation, and the best thing is it works for both genders, so any couple can try it.

If you and your partner are not that comfortable floating unsupported, you can use an inflatable mattress or any other floating water toy to help you out. Just lie with your back on the mattress to keep your head and torso out of the water, and leave your legs dangling over the end. You can also use the mattress to support a woman (or male bottom) lying on either front or back, while the other partner has sex with her by standing in the water and holding onto her legs. You'll need to be in hip-deep water for this one.

If you pass a waterfall on your trip, you can enjoy a refreshing shower before (or perhaps while) you get down and dirty. Val told me this was one her sexiest experiences: "Standing under a waterfall together—clothes and all—and feeling your nipples straightening under your T-shirt from the cold, knowing that he notices. And you feel yourself smiling. Then getting rid of the clothes." It doesn't take much imagination to figure out what happened next. Some waterfalls can also help keep you hidden from passers-by. Try to sneak between the water and the cliff.

Another classic spot for paddlers to take a break and fool around is the beach. Ever since *From Here to Eternity* made sex on the beach look *soooo* hot, almost everyone wants to give it a try. Any secluded nook close to the water's edge can make a break in your day a good chance for romance.

If you don't mind getting a bit gritty, you can simply cast off your clothes and enjoy the sand. If the beach is not so pristine, or you don't like getting sand in your bum crack, you might want to put down a barrier between you and the beach. Definitely use a barrier if you're using lubricant. Sand loves to get stuck to lube! Two jackets laid end to end should provide enough coverage, or if you're carrying a full-sized towel, that will do nicely, too. Ground sheets are another possibility. They are nice and big, but made of materials that will stick to your skin, which could be a bit uncomfortable. On the bright side, they're easy to clean off and re-pack. You could use a grass beach mat instead if you've got a bit of room in the canoe for one.

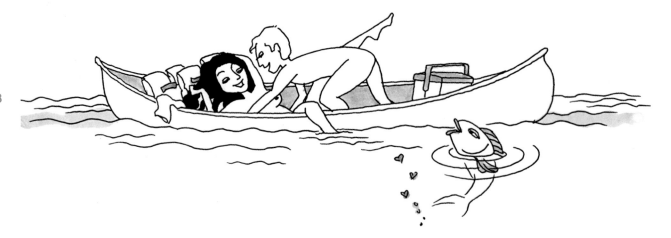

When you're picking out a beach location, make sure you have a good look around. You may be far enough from the route you were traveling not to be seen, but if there are hills or cliffs rising above you, people taking the high road could get a bird's eye view of your activities. If there is a cliff, stay as close as possible to remain hidden from sightseers above. Check for worn trails leading off the beach as well, because that's a good indication that people go there regularly.

One note of caution about beach sex: Beware of the sun. Once you strip off, you will be exposing parts of your body that don't usually see daylight. These parts can burn surprisingly quickly on a sunny beach. Either avoid beach sex during the peak midday hours, or find a shady area. You don't want to spend the rest of your camping trip with painful and peeling breasts, bums, or balls.

Once you've found an isolated spot by the water's edge, having a romp on the beach can be lots of fun. There are no constraints on positions or time. You're usually on reasonably soft ground, so it's pretty comfortable. And afterward, you can go rinse the sand off in the water and get your bathing done at the same time. Beach adventures are equally appealing at night, when you won't have to worry quite so much about hiding. Just make sure you have a flashlight with you so you can find all of your clothes and make it back to the campsite.

Sex in the water does take a little extra creativity, but it's something that you won't get to try at home (unless you have a pool), so it can make your camping trips something special to look forward to. Regardless of where you try it—on the beach, in some hot springs, or under a waterfall—take your time and indulge your senses. There's something sensual about water in nature— the rhythm of the waves, the rush of falling water, the glistening of wet rocks in the sun, the feel of saltwater drying on your skin, and the sun warming your body after a chilly dip in an isolated lake. You will not get moments like these at home.

Rocking the Boat

For some canoe trippers, making use of nature's waterbed doesn't even involve getting wet. By paddling down a smaller tributary, or hiding among some tall reeds, making love in a canoe can be a naughty perk of paddling trips.

Of course, canoes are not the most stable things in the world, so it's important to keep them balanced. Make love staying as close to the bottom as possible to keep the canoe's center of gravity low. Lay life jackets, towels, or other soft items along the bottom to provide a base on which to lie down. This is not the place to work your way through the Kama Sutra. You'll likely have to spoon or stick to the missionary position or a careful cowgirl, at least until you find your balance and discover other ways to keep from tipping over.

One couple told me about their foray into canoe-bound sexual acrobatics. "It was the first really hot summer day of the year, and I took my girlfriend on a little day trip in the canoe," says Jason. "While we were in the canoe, she told me she wanted to have sex on the water. I wasn't too sure about it—I mean, I'd never tried before—but I'd be crazy to turn down hot sex in the middle of the day, right? So we went for it." They placed life jackets along the base of the canoe, and then Jason's girlfriend slid off the front seat and lay down on the makeshift bed. Jason balanced on all fours over her, with his knees on the life jackets.

"It was all going pretty well, and soon we peeled off our swimsuits and were going at it," Jason recalls, grinning boyishly at the memory. "With the sun on my back and the motion of the water, it was amazing sex!" So amazing that after he came, he sat up, leaned against the side of the canoe, and let out a big, proud "Whoo!" of satisfaction. Big mistake.

"Before I realized what I was doing, the canoe was flipping over sideways, and we were both in the water, trying to grab our swimsuits," he says. "We lost my girlfriend's bikini top, so when we got back to the beach, she had to wear her life jacket until she could throw on a shirt in the car."

I guess there's a lesson there about securing the contents of your canoe, even your clothing. Apparently, the next time they had canoe sex, she left her bikini top tied around her neck, and they tucked their bottoms under a bungee cord. Live and learn.

One of the best variations of the missionary position for sex in a canoe is for the woman to wrap her legs around her partner's legs. This position keeps your profile very low in the canoe, so you aren't as likely to throw things off balance. It's also a great position for women, since the pelvic tilt that occurs when she stretches her legs downward causes more contact between her clitoris and her partner's pelvis, increasing her pleasure.

If there are thick reeds around you, they can help the canoe to stay stable as well. Find a marshy area where there are tall plants, close together. You'll have to use your paddles to part the reeds and really get the canoe in there among them. The reeds are great because the serve two purposes at once. They help hold the canoe in place, and they hide you from prying eyes. Before you get too far into the foreplay, give the boat a bit of a jiggle, just to see how much stability you have. The more you know from the start, the better your chances of staying afloat.

Whatever Floats Your Boat

As you can see, there are many ways to enjoy yourselves on a paddling trip. And it all starts with the old real estate cliché—"location, location, location." Choosing the spot that suits you best will make your trip more memorable. Whether you're into shooting the rapids, admiring the mirror reflection of a still lake, or exploring coastal inlets, you can find the perfect spot to be alone together.

Talk about what you're looking for in your trip before you choose where to go. How much portaging is too much? How far do you want to travel each day? Where can you find the kind of water you enjoy surrounded by gorgeous scenery?

With luck, you'll find a spot away from the crowds of other paddlers. Author Kathleen Meyer used to be a river guide and has seen many of her favorite routes become more crowded over the years. "I like to get to the more remote rivers," she says. "I find the charm in getting away from people. I like the solitude, and I don't like to have to deal with camping areas and reservations and lotteries." Often, she and her partner do trips during the winter, when they can have more space to themselves. If you're looking for that kind of solitude, you'll do well to follow her lead and seek out less popular places, or paddle off-season.

To find yourselves a romantic campsite on a paddling trip, you can't do better than small islands. You know that they'll be inaccessible to hikers, and if an island is small enough, there may only be one campsite on the whole thing. Usually, you have to be pretty rich to spend the night alone on a private island, but for paddlers, it's actually dirt cheap.

Even if you can't get your own island, you have a good chance of camping on your own little stretch of beach. Falling asleep to the sound of breaking waves makes every stroke worthwhile. Beach campsites often have lots of driftwood strewn around, which is perfect for making a cozy campfire.

Finding this kind of solitude is nearly impossible for couples in the city. So as paddlers, you are privileged to shut out the rest of the world and enjoy your time together, completely alone and uninterrupted. Not even a luxury beach resort can offer you that.

The Skinny on
Getting Rid of Crowds

" Although Geoff and I prefer to travel by foot, getting into the water can be the highlight of our trekking days. While in Corsica walking the GR 20, we got quite addicted to skinny-dipping in all the lovely rock pools that we passed. It was certainly more pleasurable than using the small, enclosed showers at the refuges, which had nowhere to hang clothes and slime on the floor from soap.

In the weeks leading up to our trip, we had been swimming naked in the River Cam to get ourselves acclimatized to cold water. (Although Geoff often worried about the pike in the river when swimming in the buff!)

On our last day of walking, we came to what would be the last rock pool of the trip. We were both eager to get in and have a final dip, but there were a lot of walkers about at this time, dipping their feet and generally just admiring the views. After a while, we began to get restless wishing these walkers would go so we could get on with our skinny-dipping.

We started to undress, thinking they might get the hint. In fact, Geoff stripped right down to his undies. A few people started to wander off, but there were still many hanging around. So Geoff said to me, "This is how to get rid of them." And with that, he stood up, took his undies off, and plunged into the depths. I have never seen people move so fast. **"**

—Sally Kelly is a walker, blogger, and skinny-dipper from King's Lynn in the United Kingdom.

Chapter 8:

HOLDING HANDS

While Backpacking

I'm a small person. Really small. Like 5 feet tall, honest. So to me, the idea of carrying around all of my gear and supplies for multiple days over miles and miles of uneven trails—well, it sounded pretty hard, and definitely not very romantic. But I decided to give it a try. The lure of wandering deep into the woods and spending the night in complete isolation with my man was enough inspiration to get me to pick up a backpack and follow him into the unknown.

The first day, I thought I might die. Not only was my pack too heavy, it kept throwing me off balance on the hills. I was sure I was going to end up on my back, stuck like an upside-down beetle in the middle of the trail, legs and arms wiggling fruitlessly as I tried to right myself. Lesson number one: Don't pack like my boyfriend. Women need to put the heaviest items near the bottom of their packs, closer to their center of gravity (men do better with the weight near the top).

The second day, I started getting the hang of it and thought I might just survive after all. And by my next trip, I was actually looking forward to it. Why the change of heart? The backcountry was incredibly peaceful and inspiring, in a way that no drive-in campsite could match. The silence of our surroundings at night created an intensity between us that I'd never felt. But I also loved the confidence I gained and accomplishment I felt at getting up a trail I once thought unsurpassable. That made me feel pretty sexy, too.

Even if you start out like I was and can't imagine carrying yourself that far, let alone a loaded backpack, keep an open mind. Like any new form of exercise, you'll just have to work your way up from short, level tracks to…well, the sky is pretty much the limit. Nepal, anyone? If you're starting to think it all sounds too tough for you, just remember that a guy with two amputated legs has climbed Mt. Everest, so don't be such a wuss! It will all be worth it when you and your partner reach your spectacular campsite with nobody else in sight. Alone at last!

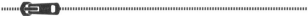

Silky-Smooth **Snuggles**

❝ My boyfriend and I go backpacking together a lot. Just short trips, mostly on weekends. We always zip our sleeping bags together so we can snuggle up. We saw in some stores they had silk sleeping bag liners, and they looked really nice and comfortable, but that meant having separate little bags inside our big one, which kind of defeated the purpose.

So when we went on a holiday in Thailand, I got all excited when I realized how cheap it is to buy silk there. I got a big piece of wonderful, soft silk (it's bright blue) and found a woman with an old sewing machine working on the sidewalk. I asked her to sew it into a sack for us.

Now we've got our own custom-made double sleeping bag liner made of gorgeous Thai silk. It's so nice to sleep in that sometimes we even use it a home. Then we can pretend we're camping any night we want! **❞**

—PT

Romantic Gestures in the Wilderness

Slogging over a trail with 30 pounds or more on your back may not sound romantic, but romance is all about your attitude. You can be romantic while hiking through 15 miles of mud, if you set your mind to it. Or you can turn a sunset stroll along the beach into a total drag by deciding you're having a bad time.

One of the easiest ways to keep things romantic is right in the chapter's title—hold hands. It may sound cheesy, but it's a small gesture that makes you feel closer. If it's all a bit too cliché for you, how about touching your partner somewhere else? There should be some shoulder you can reach, or even a teasing bum grope might be possible, depending on how much stuff is hanging off your partner's pack. Your trip is about being together, so keep making contact in case your partner has forgotten you're there. And don't ignore the direct approach. If you stop for a drink of water, lean in and go for a kiss, too. You can never have too many kiss breaks, as far as I'm concerned.

It's easy to fall into a silent, marching pattern while you hike. So make an effort to share what's on your mind. You don't have to chatter nonstop (you went out there for some peace and quiet, after all), but when you notice something interesting, spot an animal, or find a nice view, include your partner. You're out there to share an experience, so share!

If talking about the scenery doesn't get you going, how about talking out your fantasies? Just like paddling, hiking is a perfect time to let your imagination run wild. Couples therapist Esther Perel finds that couples with an imagination can play out those fantasy roles anywhere, but it can be helpful to have a setting that matches. "Roles are products of the imagination," she says. "Some people may find it easier to switch into a role when nature heightens it. It's easier to be Tarzan with trees around. It's easier to be a pirate if there's water."

It's easier to let your fantasy life take over when there's nobody else around to pass judgment, so a secluded trail is the perfect place to tell your partner about a fantasy you've had. If you're feeling really creative, you can plan an entire trip around your fantasy scenario. You could search for a lost, ancient civilization, and maybe the tribal god-king forces the two of you to perform for him. Or you could be two of the first settlers in the New World looking for a place to build your homestead. (Just don't get carried away and start clearing the forest!) Your new, rustic home definitely needs to be christened. Build a story to match your setting, or choose a setting that works with your story. Be detailed about it. Is it something you could role play later that night?

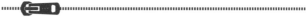

Going the Distance for Love

❝ My husband and I met at Cornell University. His roommate and my roommate were a couple, and so we got together through them. But we were both into camping and they weren't, so we ended up going on little backpacking trips around upstate New York together. Then over the summers, we both had jobs in New York City, so we started doing weekend trips on the Appalachian Trail.

By the time we graduated, we'd done all 88 miles of the trail in New York. To celebrate, we decided to take a vacation and hike the beginning of the AT in Georgia. We spent five days backpacking, ending up at Springer Mountain, the start of the trail.

When we got to the trailhead my boyfriend said, "We've done over 100 miles of the trail. Now, we have just 2000 miles to go." I told him at the rate we were going, that was going to take the rest of our lives, and he said, "I hope so." Then he reached into his pocket and pulled out a box with a diamond ring, and asked me to walk with him for the rest of our lives! When I stopped crying, I said yes. By the way, we're up to 320 miles now. ❞

—ST

Here's another little game to help you keep the conversation interesting. It's called "The First Time." Take turns presenting each other with the opening to a story. It should always start with "The first time I…" and then your partner will have to finish it truthfully. Here are some examples to get you started:

The first time I French kissed…
The first time I cooked dinner for a date…
The first time I spent the night at a lover's house…
The first time I met you…

You get the picture. This is a great way to recapture the early days of your relationship if you've been together for a long time. And if you're in a new relationship, it's a nice way to get to know each other better.

The best time to add some quality cuddling to your day is when you take your packs off for a break. What a relief! The euphoria of getting that weight off your back should have you feeling friendlier already. Give your partner a little shoulder rub to ease those stiff muscles (a nice partner will give you one back!). Even if you're all sweaty, it's a good time for a hug and a smooch.

Selecting Secluded Trails

Popular hiking trails can seem like little interstates, with people rambling up and down all day. Sometimes I even feel like I need a passing lane to get through the traffic. It's great to see so many people enjoying the outdoors, but it's a little depressing, too. I go backpacking to get away from the crowds and feel like I'm surrounded by nature, not to hang out with dozens of other hikers. But I have to admit that it's usually my own fault (or my partner's, let's blame him, OK?). When we choose a trail based on how quickly we can get there from the city, or how conveniently it loops for a weekend trip, it's obvious that a lot of other people are going to be choosing the same trail for the same reasons. So how do you throw them off the scent and get a bit of solitude?

Choosing a backpacking trail for solitude is a lot like choosing a car camping location, only it's easier because there are far fewer people spread out over a lot more space. But the same principles apply.

The first and best trick is to go off-season. This can be a bit tricky with backpacking, because it may involve going in colder weather, which means carrying heavier clothing and bulkier sleeping bags. On the flip side, you can't beat the silence of hiking on a trail in October or November. If you choose well, you'll get to see some spectacular fall colors as the leaves turn shades of red and gold. Not only that, but you'll avoid mosquito season, too. If you

carry a bit more, fall backpacking is a sure way to spend some quiet time with your partner.

If you're both hardy enough to go winter camping, you'll be even better off. Aside from a few hut-to-hut skiers, almost nobody backpacks in the winter. Plus, you'll get to see a whole new side of the wilderness that most people miss—blankets of snow covering the ground and the trees. The only sound is the creaking of your feet in the snow. The only signs of human activity are your own footprints trailing off behind you. It's like living in a Christmas card!

If going off-season doesn't work for you, it's almost as good to go mid-week. Most of us have day jobs and have to fit our backpacking into weekend outings. If you

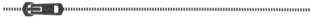

Hut-to-Hut
Hideaways

Some backpacking trips involve hiking from hut to hut, and not sleeping in a tent at all. Backcountry huts are still pretty rare in America, but they are gaining popularity, especially in the form of "yurts," round structures that are modeled on the traditional homes of Mongolian nomads. In other countries, throughout Europe, Australia, Africa, and New Zealand, camping huts are plentiful in wilderness parks.

This can be a very nice way to get around, with good shelter from rainy weather and sometimes even running water and gas stoves. The tradeoff is privacy. If you're on a popular trail, you aren't likely to get the hut to yourselves, so sex is going to be off the menu at night. If you find yourselves in a shared hut, make the most of it. Sleep side by side and snuggle close to each other. Keep your sleeping bags partially open so you can touch a little. If there isn't anyone right next to you, you can probably get away with a bit of playful fondling, and some naughty whispers in the dark.

have some vacation days to use, try taking a trip during the week. You can check out a longer trail that you normally don't have time for, or maybe one that's a little farther away from where you live. Unless it's on everyone's to-do list (like the Grand Canyon or New Zealand's Milford Track), you'll run into very few people from Sunday evening to Friday afternoon.

Try to avoid those places that will always be busy because they're convenient or well-known for their beauty. Why compete with everyone else when all you want is to enjoy a romantic escape? Get some good maps of the area and check out the options. Are there parks you've never visited? Are there less-used entrances to the parks?

You'll probably need good topographical maps of the areas where you're planning to go. So choose a park and have a look at the route you'd like to take. Is it hike-in access only, or will paddlers be able to get there? How many backcountry campsites are there, and how far apart are they? Does more than one trail lead to the same location? The more ways there are to access a spot, the more people will probably be there. If you're determined not to see another soul while you're backpacking, you're going to have to do your homework and find somewhere really hard to reach. You can also find out about crowds and busy seasons by talking with local rangers and reading guidebooks about your intended trail.

Then again, privacy can be overrated. For Wyoming native Erica, being on a well-traveled trail actually led her to love. She grew up hiking on the Continental Divide Trail with her family, so when her mother passed away from breast cancer, she and her sister decided to pay her tribute by volunteering to do trail maintenance for two weeks during the summer. She found the experience of giving back to this trail she had enjoyed for so long really rewarding. And it gave her a whole new perspective on a wilderness she thought she knew.

"While we were there, we spent time with the other volunteers, one of which was this really nice guy from

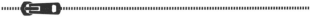

Signs You Might Have Chosen *a Bad Trail for Romance*

You reach your campsite after a six-hour hike, just as an entire Boy Scout troop is pulling up right beside you in their canoes.

People passing the other way just shake their heads and say, "Good luck."

Halfway through your first day, you pass a McDonalds.

As you're hiking, you spot a helicopter hovering nearby, and it flies away after winching up a hiker on a stretcher.

You keep coming across signs that say: Landslide—detour.

Your map has the trail labeled as the "Mosquito Swamp Trail."

Your waterfront campsite actually looks a lot like that moon where Yoda lived.

You step in bear droppings five times in one day.

You see a house made of gingerbread, or meet a talking wolf.

Montana. Not just nice, but super-cute!" Erica says. "We kept in touch afterward, and eventually I moved out to Montana to live with him." So if there was any doubt about good deeds paying off, there's your proof! They look for less-populated spots to camp together now, but they still do volunteer trail maintenance once a year.

Another Montana resident, author Kathleen Meyer, believes you can make the most of any camping location. If the summit trails are too crowded, why not appreciate natural beauty on a different scale? "Those long vistas of grandeur that you get at high points are so glorious, but there are places where you can just sit and look at the vegetation and the rock formations at your feet and see

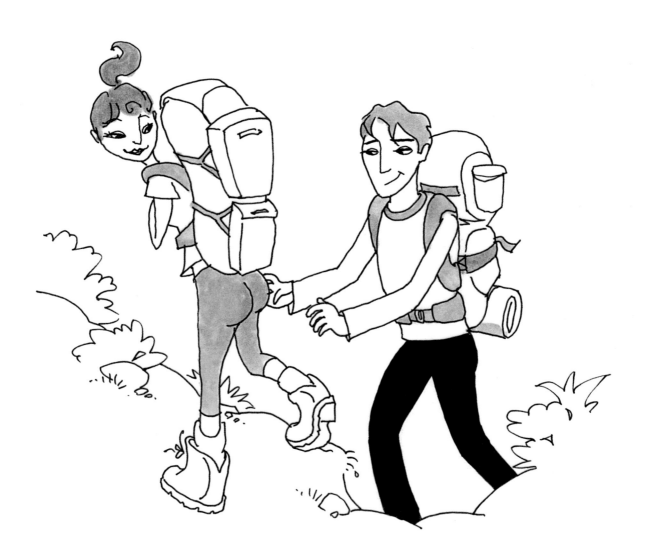

the tiniest little community," she says. "I find it just as inspiring." Sometimes by altering your expectations just a little, you can make it a lot easier to find a trail that meets those expectations.

Frontcountry Foreplay

If you're backpacking along a trail that's not too busy, you may be able to take advantage of your distance from "polite society" even before you get to your campsite. Heather and her husband once were on such an isolated trail in Arizona's Sierra Ancha Wilderness, that they took their clothes off and did it right there on the trail.

For most of us, the trail itself is too risky, but you may be able to find enough seclusion in the bush to have a quick tryst. Just make sure that you are far enough from the trail that other users passing by can't see you, but close enough that you can find your way back in your post-coital euphoria.

My friend Maria was innocently hiking with her boyfriend and another couple along a lakeside trail in the Rockies one day, when they discovered a couple who hadn't quite traveled far enough off the trail. "We suddenly saw two blonde heads pop up," Maria says. "They were lying down by the lakeside in the grass. The man put on his shirt in a very hurried way. The woman still had a tank top on and kept her back turned to us." Maria thinks she was at least as embarrassed as they were.

If you find a soft, grassy area, you can just throw down your jackets and make love on the ground, and if the grass is nice and high, it will shield you from sight. Wooded areas also make good hiding places, but it's a bit harder to find a nice, soft piece of ground. You can always put down a sleeping pad to protect you from the tree roots. If you're close to the trail, try to find a place above it not below it, or people will be able to look down at you.

Since you're going to be surrounded by trees in most cases, why not use them to help keep you off the ground?

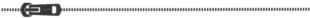

The Foggiest Idea

66 My wife and I were on a four-day backpacking trip in New Zealand's Tararua Mountains, staying in huts at night. It was a long weekend, and the huts were crowded. There was nowhere to be alone at night, and no way to do anything on the bunks without a bunch of people seeing and hearing us. It was a bit of a drag, but it was an amazing trail, so we just decided it was worth sacrificing our privacy.

One night, the hut was so crowded, we decided to skip our hot breakfast the next day and just get out of there early. We were the first ones out the door at 7 a.m. Outside there was a thick mist, and we set off along the trail.

After about half an hour of walking and not seeing another soul, we left the trail and went behind a stand of trees. The foggy weather hid us from sight completely, so we quickly dropped our packs and undressed to have sex standing against the trees. Shrouded by the mist, it was an almost magical experience. There was steam rising from our bodies and mixing with the fog. It was unreal. That made up for all of the sexless nights! 99

—GD

If hugging a tree is good, then having sex against one must be really, really good, right? There are a few different positions you can try. The man can back the woman against the tree and hold her under her buttocks, lifting her legs off the ground. This one's for strong guys only, because if you lose your grip, your partner's back will scrape against the tree, and that might make her a tad angry.

You may find it easier to avoid any accidental abrasions if you are both facing the tree, and the woman puts her hands on the trunk to brace herself while the man enters from behind. If you can find a tree with a strong, low branch, try having the woman lean over it. If the branch isn't too twiggy, this is probably the most comfortable position.

Off-trail warning: The main thing to watch out for when you wander into the bush for some action is any kind of irritating plant. Poison ivy or poison oak can turn a sexy romp in the woods into days of discomfort, especially if they come into contact with your privates (even if you're into pain, this is probably not the kind of pain you're looking for). Know what these plants look like and check the ground before you get naked and rub up against them. While you're at it, make sure you aren't too close to anything with thorns. They can spoil the mood pretty fast, too.

Off-trail sex isn't everyone's idea of a great time. If it seems a bit much, or you've got too much ground to cover to take a big break for sex, then take it down a notch. Sneak off the trail and make out instead, like a couple of high school students sneaking away from the big game. Keep your clothes on, but get your hands up under your partner's shirt, or, better yet, down your partner's pants! Give each other a quick thrill without having to drop your drawers in the open.

Building a Desirable Campsite

After a long day of backpacking and getting in the mood for a wonderfully remote night with your partner, you finally arrive at your backcountry campsite. Your next challenge is to turn a patch of dirt into your private paradise. Setting up a love nest in the wilderness isn't difficult, but it takes some thought. After all, on a back-packing trip you probably have only one night in each spot, so you've got to get it right the first time.

It all begins in the planning stages of your trip, especially if you have to book your campsites ahead of time. Make sure you've got a good map of the place you're going and that all of the campsites are marked on it. It's hard to tell what a site will be like from the little dot on a map, but there are a few things you can figure out. First of all, is it the only site in the area? You don't want to be in the middle of a cluster of campsites where you could have unwanted neighbors. If it's the only site around, you'll probably get to spend the night by yourselves.

You may also be able to tell how close it is to a beach or a riverbank. This is good for practical considerations like getting water for cooking and washing, but it also lets you know if you might be able to go for a private swim at some point. Is the water out of sight of the main trail? Is your campsite the closest one to a lake? If so, you could think about skinny-dipping. Or maybe you'd like to arrive in time to have a walk along the beach once you set up camp.

Find the sites that look the most appealing, and then use the map and any trail guides you have to figure out how far you want to walk each day. In the end, there's no point in finding the perfect campsite if you won't get there until midnight.

Some parks allow you to camp anywhere, not just on designated sites. Now you've really got options! Make sure you have a topographic map, so you can find flat areas to pitch your tent at your destination. You'll still want to be close to some water, so you can use it for cooking and replenishing your drinking supplies. Get a general idea of where you'd like to spend the night, but be sure to arrive there well before sunset. If your perfect spot ends up being not-so-perfect when you get there, you'll need time to find a back-up. But having the whole park available to you means you'll definitely be able to find somewhere you can spend the night completely alone.

Once you're actually at your campsite, it's time to set it up in the best possible way for your night of love and solitude. Here are some things to look for: somewhere to set up the tent that's flat and sheltered from the wind, some good trees to hang up your hammock if you've brought one, a place to make a campfire if they're allowed (and some dead wood to burn), a nice place for a walk

Paddling vs. **Backpacking**

❝ We used to do a lot of kayaking trips. My husband is such a strong paddler that I hardly had to do any work at all! But recently we started backpacking, too, and I've noticed some of the advantages of it. When we're paddling, we have to experience the same things at the same time because we're pretty much stuck together all day.

Backpacking allows us to be two individuals. I love the scenery we get to see when we're kayaking, but it's like that's the big picture, and backpacking is the close-up. You can get in there and explore more on your feet. One of us can slow down if there's something we want to take a closer look at. We can spend time right beside each other, or have a bit of space.

It's up to us and what moods we're in. If he wants to take on a big climb at full speed, he can go for it and wait for me at the top. I don't want to stop kayaking, but I'm really glad I decided to give backpacking a try because it's opened up a whole new world for me. **❞**

—WJ

or a swim nearby, and places where you'll be invisible to anyone walking the same trail you came in on.

It sounds like a tall order, doesn't it? Luckily, most backcountry sites have most of those things, if not all of them. Whether you can light a campfire will depend on the recent weather and local rules, but most designated campsites have flat tent areas, a sheltered location, and water nearby. Now it's up to you to set up camp to make the most of it.

Before you set up your tent, look for animal tracks. You won't have a very good time in there if you realize in the middle of the night that you're parked along a wildlife highway. If your tent is between their homes and their drinking water, you could have a lot of unwelcome visitors, so steer clear of places with visible tracks or droppings. The other thing that can spoil your night is flooding, so don't set up your tent in an area where water will pool in if it's raining. Otherwise, your tent is your camping bedroom, so put it somewhere comfy and out of the way.

If you've brought a hammock along, make sure the trees you use to support it are sturdy enough to handle the weight of both people at once. Later in this chapter, I describe all kinds of fun activities you can use your hammock for, but you definitely don't want to break the trees!

Once you've got things set up, walk back to the trail. How visible is your campsite to other backpackers? Where are the best areas for staying out of sight? If you decide to fool around outside the tent, it's helpful to know ahead of time whether there's a chance of being seen by other people.

Dinner is a major event at the end of a hard day of backpacking. Try to give it the attention it deserves. As I mentioned in Chapter 4, the setting for your meal can be as important as what you're eating. Take a stroll around your campsite and see where the best view is. Can you see mountains, a lake, a coastline, or some other amazing scenery? Make that your backdrop when it comes time to sit and eat. If there's no obvious feature to look at, try to face the setting sun. A flat rock or smooth log can be a comfortable seat so you don't have to eat on the ground. If you're hiding from rain, set up a tarp to cook and eat under so you don't have to be shut inside the tent right away.

Boinking in the Backcountry

Your campsite is full of opportunities for sex, and because you're in the backcountry, you won't have to worry about hiding inside your tent. By now, you've had a chance to

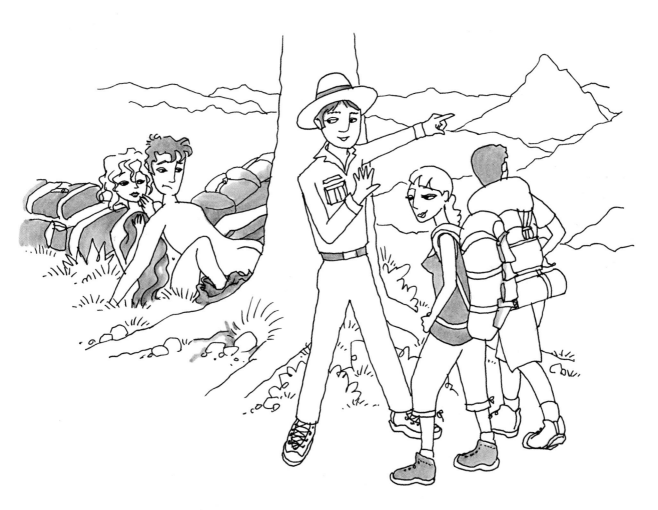

look around and find a good spot, out of view of the trails. The next step? Just do it!

But let's say you want to create a little ambiance first. I think campfires are insanely romantic, and I know I'm not alone here. I love the smell of burning wood, the gorgeous light they create that gives everything a soft, orange glow, and best of all, the warmth of sitting close to a fire. I'm all for taking advantage of that warmth to dispense with extra (or all) clothing. Again, a couple of jackets or a ground sheet will be helpful to keep you out of the dirt. If fireside sex is too adventurous for you, it's still a great location for kissing, cuddling, and petting. Then you can slip into the tent to get down to some serious love-making.

Getting down and dirty on the ground just doesn't appeal to some people. If you want to elevate things a bit, look for a large, flat rock. Some campsites are situated near large rocks so that campers can use as the rock as a "table" for preparing and eating food. Throw a sleeping pad on top of the rock, and you've got yourselves a raised bed. This gives you more options when it comes to sexual positions (see "Setting the Table," mentioned in Chapter 6), while at the same time keeping you away from dirt, roots, and bugs. Large rocks and fallen logs around the campsite are also helpful when it comes to oral sex. The receiving partner can sit on the edge of the rock or log and let the giver kneel in front. Nature (and the Park Service) provides plenty of great sexual aids that you don't have to pack in with you.

If you've got enough space in your pack, however, perhaps the best sexual toy you can bring is a hammock. Get a two-person hammock and tie it up securely, 'cause this baby's gonna swing! The only rule: Don't fall out.

It's not as easy as it sounds. If you try a basic position like missionary, you'll discover that with the hammock's droopy shape, it's hard to brace yourself. But there are some positions that work really well in a hammock. Spooning is excellent because the side-to-side motion

of thrusting in this position will also get the hammock swinging. Or you can lie on your sides facing each other, and the woman can wrap her top leg around her partner's lower back. If you can keep yourselves balanced in the hammock, you might just be ready to attempt sex in a canoe. If you're up for a bit of fun, have the woman (or man in a same-sex couple) lie face down lying across the hammock. The man then enters from behind, holds her legs, and swings her toward his hips, so that the thrusting is actually done by the hammock.

Returning to Civilized Society

I can't help it. When I return from a backpacking trip, I'm always really happy—and not just from the great outdoor loving. There's that sense of accomplishment that puts a smile on my face every time. But there's also a sense of deflation as we face the long drive back to the city in smelly clothes, munching on leftover GORP. But a bit of advanced planning can finish off any trip in style.

I suggest packing a "return to civilization kit" and stowing it in the car. Here's what to bring:

A plastic basin or bucket, water, soap, shampoo and conditioner, deodorant, razor, and shaving cream

A change of clothes for each of you—something comfortable but attractive, too

A small but nice snack like fresh fruit, cookies, or whatever you will be missing by then

And here's the clincher:

Make dinner reservations at a nice restaurant that's on your way home.

Now you've got everything you need to get cleaned up and feeling human again, and you don't have to worry about making dinner when you get home. Try to find a nice country inn near the park so you don't have far to go for your dinner stop. This will get you tons of brownie points if your partner is not usually a "roughing it" sort of person, and you want to show your appreciation. And don't you both deserve a nice reward for all of your efforts over the trip?

Backpacking trips can be whatever the two of you want them to be. From a couple of hours walking into a park for the weekend, right up to thru-hiking a long-distance trail and living in the wilderness for months. Either way, you'll probably find the time you spend doing it is more rewarding than just about any other part of your relationship. There's no doubt that couples bond when they're backpacking, and while you might not get along perfectly 100 percent of the time, you'll probably find your relationship has grown stronger by the time you reach home. In the end, getting back to the box of your bedroom might not seem too confining after you've learned the secrets of making love in a tent.

Appendix 1:

THE MOST ROMANTIC CAMPSITES

in North America

By now you've probably got a pretty good idea of how you want your next camping trip to go. The only decision left is *where* to go. Americans are spoiled for choice, so this entire section is filled with ideas for romantic camping getaways in North America.

I know that it's tempting to go for the biggies—the places you always hear about. I personally couldn't resist the lure of the Grand Canyon. I absolutely needed to hike to the bottom and experience this world-famous icon from the inside out. As you can guess, a lot of people have the same idea. But when I hiked into the Grand Canyon with a guide and two other backpackers, we didn't see another person the whole day. Impossible, you say? Not at all! You just have to put down the glossy brochure and get away from the "usual" route.

We hiked down the South Canyon Trail, a little-used route that follows a dry river valley into Marble Canyon, and eventually meets the Colorado River. We camped on a small, comfortable beach near a waterfall called Vaseys Paradise. It was a tough hike—too tough for my level of experience at the time—but with the help of our guide, I made it down in six grueling, sweaty hours. Did I mention that I did this during an unusual spring heat wave? I'd tell you how hot it was, but we reached the top of the thermometer, so I'm not really sure.

Even without a guide, you can find plenty of ways to avoid the crowds. If you have to do the biggies, try to do them off-season, mid-week, or using lesser-known routes. I've included ideas for seeing some classic biggies in this appendix, but everyone has their own must-see list, so don't limit yourself to what's here.

If you don't have a list of places you absolutely have to see, then you'll have a lot less trouble finding spots for a private, romantic getaway. Just invest in some good maps and do a bit of exploring. Or use the ideas in this appendix and the next one to get you started.

Northwest US

The **Strawberry Mountain Wilderness** in Oregon's Malheur National Forest offers visitors jagged peaks, flowering meadows, and abundant wildlife. And with a name like "Strawberry Mountain," it even sounds romantic! The nearest town is John Day, which you've probably never heard of, but with 100 miles of hiking trails through some spectacular mountain scenery, it's worth finding. And, of course, there's no need to worry about crowds, unless you consider the deer population a problem. If backpacking in the mountains sounds too strenuous, you can enjoy the trails as dayhikes from the Strawberry Campground instead. **More Information:** Strawberry Mountain Wilderness at 541-575-3000; www.fs.fed.us/r6/Malheur.

Idaho's **Sawtooth Mountains** offer that irresistible rugged skyline that draws people from all over the country. Hiking below these spectacular peaks is so popular that it can require booking campsites far in advance during the peak summer season. The place is just loaded with backpackers, paddlers, and rock climbers looking for a piece of the action. At higher altitudes, the snow can last into June, which makes the crowding even worse over the short summer season.

For a more remote and peaceful experience in the Sawtooth, try backpacking the **Queen's River Loop**. You'll get to see the rugged peaks, mountain lakes, and flowering fields that everyone loves so much, but without all of the other people. Plus, you'll get the unusual experience of hiking through a rocky chasm for a whole different perspective. **More Information:** Sawtooth Wilderness at 208-737-3200; www.fs.fed.us/r4/sawtooth/recreation/wildernessindex.htm.

Glacier National Park, Montana, and **Waterton Lakes National Park**, Alberta, offer a cross-border sampling of the Rockies that's got something for everyone. Car campers can choose from 1000 sites on 10 campgrounds, so the odds of finding a bit of privacy, especially

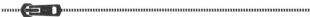

The Biggies:
Yellowstone National Park

Yellowstone is the granddaddy of all national parks. It covers a huge 3,472 square miles and is visited by almost 3 million people each year.

But here's another, less-known statistic about Yellowstone—of all those annual visitors crowding the park, less than 1 percent of them bother to get a backcountry permit and spend a night in the park interior. So if you're up for a bit of exploration, Yellowstone's 1000 miles or so of trails will be anything but crowded.

One area to check out is the park's southwest corner. The **Bechler** area features lots of waterfalls that create lovely rainbows. Flowering meadows are a visual treat, and you can indulge yourselves in a romantic soak in nature's hot tubs. It's illegal to bathe in any of the park's hot pools, but where they empty into rivers, you're welcome to soak in the warmth. Sounds like a romantic trip to me! And if you really must, you can always stop off to see Old Faithful before or after your interior trip. **More Information:** Yellowstone National Park at 307-344-7381; www.nps.gov/yell.

mid-week, are pretty good. The parks also offer some of the most spectacular road trips in the country for mountain scenery. For those who want to stretch their legs, there are about 700 miles of trails to explore. If you're looking for solitude, head for the southern part of Glacier National Park. Spotting grizzly bears is not unusual here, so make some noise while you're walking. For paddlers, there are also a lot of options here. Glacial runoff rivers provide whitewater for you adventurous couples, and a number of lakes give you flatter, more relaxing options. **More Information:** Glacier National Park at 406-888-7800; www.nps.gov/glac, or Waterton Lakes National Park at 403-859-2224; www.pc.gc.ca/pn-np/ab/waterton.

Northeast US

The **Allagash Wilderness Waterway** winds through vast private timber forests in Maine. A hundred years ago, Henry David Thoreau was guided through the area and found it awe-inspiring. It's our collective good luck that not much has changed along the Allagash since then. The waterway is a protected wilderness area, although there are constant battles between conservationists and those who would like to improve public access. You can still find yourselves completely removed from civilization as you paddle the 92 miles of rivers, ponds, lakes, and streams. A lot of visitors claim that they see more moose than people on their trips! **More Information:** Allagash Wilderness Waterway at 207-941-4014; www.state.me.us.

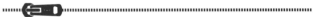

The Biggies:
Adirondacks

The Adirondacks are a magnet for New York hiking enthusiasts. Every summer, the most popular trails are peppered with dayhikers and backpackers looking to spend some quality time in the mountains. That can make it tough to feel like you're really enjoying nature, and it sure hampers your chances of seeing any wildlife. So forget about the trails that have been everyone's favorites for decades. By getting away from the most impressive mountains and classic hikes, you'll be able to ditch the crowd. Call it sacrificing a bit of altitude for a lot more solitude.

The **Siamese Ponds Wilderness** is a great example. It offers more than 175 acres of low mountains (up to about 3,400 feet), rivers, and dozens of ponds and lakes (36 to be exact!). Keep an eye out, and you may get to see otters, beavers, and loons, and maybe even a bald eagle. **More Information:** Adirondack Park at 518-891-4050; www.apa.state.ny.us.

I can't ignore the **Boundary Waters Canoe Area Wilderness** in Minnesota, even though it is one of the most visited wilderness areas in the country. With 1200 miles of canoe routes, you can definitely get away from the crowds here. The park has 73 different entry points, and a quota system for permits, so that even the most popular places aren't horribly overused. The US Forest Service compiles visitation data every year, so you can check with them to see which routes are the least used and the most likely to give you privacy.

One area that seems to be away from the hoards is the end of the Gunflint region, including Seagull Lake, Alpine Lake, Rog Lake, and Jasper Lake. Or try the Poplar Lake area: The adjoining lakes are smaller than most, with an abundance of lovely scenery. You may have to sacrifice the convenience of nearby facilities, but who needs facilities when you've got each other? **More Information:** Boundary Waters Canoe Area Wilderness at 218-626-4300; www.fs.fed.us/r9/forests/superior/bwcaw.

Southwest US

If you think that your only options for getting outdoors in Arizona involve canyons and deserts, it's time to head east. The **Blue Range Primitive Area,** near the New Mexico border, leads you through actual forests full of pine, spruce, and aspen, and even reliable sources of water so you don't have to hike in carrying a multiday supply. The Blue Range also features about 200 miles of trails to choose from, so privacy is plentiful. There are a lot of snakes here, so it isn't the best choice for those of you with phobias of legless creatures, but if you can get past the reptile population, you could also be rewarded with a glimpse of black bears, elk, beavers, wild turkeys, bighorn sheep, and mountain lions. And skyward you should keep your eyes peeled for a peregrine falcon or a bald eagle. **More Information:** Blue Range Primitive Area at 928-333-4301; www.fs.fed.us/r3/asnf.

The **Ruby Mountains** in Nevada sound pretty enticing, don't they? Sadly, you won't find any actual rubies there.

The mountains got their name from the other red gemstone, garnet. I guess the first people to find them needed to brush up on their gemstone identification skills! I can't vouch for your chances of finding any jewels during your stay, but at least you can enjoy some amazing mountain scenery while you search. This 100-mile-long range is a great place to get some space to yourselves and do a bit of backpacking with a lot of romance.

The only place in the Rubies that normally sees crowds is the road-accessible Lamoille Canyon. You could see as many as 100 cars parked in the lot there on a busy day, but rest assured that most are just dayhikers. After your first couple of hours on the trail, they'll simply disappear. If you want a guarantee of quiet trails, use the trailhead at Soldier Canyon instead. No more than 10 cars can park there, so there's no chance of a crowd anywhere in sight.

The 40-mile **Ruby Crest Trail** is the main backpacking route through the range, but it has plenty of side trails, so you can make your own routes and see as few people as you like. If you're really determined to avoid any chance of running into other backpackers, you could try bushwhacking off-trail to some of the less-accessible lakes. **More Information:** Ruby Mountains Wilderness at 775-331-6444; www.fs.fed.us/r4/htnf/districts/ruby_mountain.

For a good taste of the rugged desert scenery the southwest is so famous for, take a trip to **Canyonlands National Park** in Utah. You will find few other visitors if you have the experience and independent spirit to head for the Maze district of the park. As the name suggests, this area has a maze of canyon walls to explore. You'll have a tough time spending more than a day there though, since there's no source of water nearby. Perhaps a day of solitude in the Maze could be followed up with a couple more exploring the more accessible (and better supplied) areas of the park. **More Information:** Canyonlands National Park at 435-719-2313; www.nps.gov/cany.

If you're into car camping and want to check out the Sierra Nevada mountains, you'll have a good chance

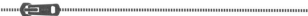

The Biggies:
Grand Canyon

This may be the biggie of all biggies. I've wanted to go ever since I watched Wyle E. Coyote plunging off the side again and again when I was 3! (I don't know if that was supposed to be the Grand Canyon, but my 3-year-old imagination thought it was.) Most people settle for a day trip from Las Vegas, where they crowd along viewpoints taking pictures and trying to wrap their heads around the sheer size of this thing.

If you plan it right, you can get a spectacular view of the canyon without the crowds. I stayed at a fantastic car-camping site in **Kaibab National Forest** that overlooks the canyon. And I mean it really overlooks the canyon! If you pitched your tent too close to the edge, you could have a nasty accident getting up during the night to pee. Best of all, there was nobody else in sight. All we had to do was reserve the site during the less-crowded period in early spring. If you've got just a single romantic bone in your body, you'll positively melt when you have dinner watching the sun set over the Grand Canyon. This biggie's worth it! **More Information:** Kaibab National Forest at 928-635-8200; www.fs.fed.us/r3/kai.

As I mentioned earlier, there are also some pretty remote trails leading down into the Grand Canyon if you're up for a serious hike. Just stay away from the masses of rim-to-rim hikers on the Bright Angel Trail, and you'll be free to quietly admire one of nature's wonders from within.

of finding something that suits you in one of the 40 campgrounds in **Stanislaus National Forest.** Most of the campgrounds have a 14-day limit but don't require advance bookings. Some popular destinations will fill up, particularly on long weekends, but with more than 1000 sites, you should be able to find a nice spot somewhere.

Get a map of the forest and decide where you'd like to be. Fishing in one of the mountain lakes? Exploring trails on dayhikes? Find the campground that is best suited to the activities you have in mind. Remember, the harder it is to reach, the more privacy you'll get, so invest some time and effort and you'll be richly rewarded. There are no electric hookups at any of the campgrounds, so at the very least you can be guaranteed an RV-free experience. **More Information:** Stanislaus National Forest at 209-532-3671; www.fs.fed.us/r5/Stanislaus.

Southeast US

A lot of people in the eastern part of the US are drawn to the impressive length and reputation of the Appalachian Trail. But most of us will never have the time (or energy!) to tackle the whole 2,100 miles, and the sections that are most accessible from major cities can get crowded. As an alternative, think about hiking the **Foothills Trail,** which bridges the borders of South Carolina and North Carolina. At 86 miles, it is a long enough through-hike for you goal-oriented types who may not have the luxury of taking an extended leave from work.

As you can guess from the name, the Foothills Trail doesn't get into the highest parts of the Appalachians, but stays in the Cherokee Foothills. For that reason alone, a lot of people overlook it, but this trail offers gorgeous scenery and a chance to enjoy it in solitude. The vast number of waterfalls along the trail makes it one of the most romantic long-distance backpacking trips in the country. There are private companies at the ends of the trail to shuttle you back to your car, too, so there's no need to bring two vehicles. **More Information:** Foothills Trail at 866-224-9339; www.foothillstrail.org.

Louisiana doesn't have much of a reputation for wilderness excursions. Mostly people think of it as flat and swampy, but there is some great camping to be done in the state. Why not check out the **Wild Azalea Trail,** a 31-mile route that's anything but flat. There are at least five ecosystems represented along the trail, including pine-covered hills and some of Louisiana's famous bayous. You'll find cypress trees down low, then hickory, oak, and dogwood on your way up to the pines.

If you're looking for a romantic spot for car camping, how could you miss out on **Valentine Lake** campground? The facilities are pretty basic, but you can access the Wild Azalea Trail from a connecting path at the campground and explore it on a dayhike. The trail has several road access points, so you can also get dropped off somewhere along the way and hike your way back to the camp-ground. That gives you a chance to see more of the trail without having to backtrack.

For backpackers, the whole trail can be completed in three days, and there are a number of tent sites along the way, some of which are very close to water sources.

The Biggies:
Great Smoky Mountains

The Smokies are legendary for their awesome beauty, and as part of the Appalachian Trail, they see more than 10 million visitors per year—more than any other national park in the US. Don't be daunted by the numbers, as there are still places within Great Smoky Mountains National Park where you can enjoy the splendor without the traffic.

The best way to avoid the crowds is to get away from the Appalachian Trail. Try visiting the park's southeast corner, where less-used trails offer you a chance for a roman-tic weekend. The **Spruce Mountain Loop** is a two-day backpacking trip with a wide variety of terrain, including a grassy valley, spruce and fir forests higher up, and even the remains of a pioneer homestead. So find your own pioneer spirit, and head for the majestic Smoky Mountains. **More Information:** Great Smoky Mountains National Park at 865-436-1200; www.nps.gov/grsm.

The trail is pretty quiet all year long, but the most solitude (and fewest mosquitoes) can be found in the winter. With all of the major water crossings bridged, you don't have to worry about cold, wet feet, either. **More Information:** Wild Azalea Trail at 318-473-7160; www.fs.fed.us/r8/kisatchie; or Valentine Lake Campground at 318-793-9427.

Alaska

Misty Fjords National Monument is a paddler's paradise. As the name suggests, the weather can be wet in this area, so bring good rain gear to keep warm and dry. You can book cabins to sleep in through the Forest Service, which is nice if the weather is wet. You'll have a good chance of seeing whales and orcas, not to mention bears, on fishing expeditions. Hiking trails to nearby lakes make a nice break from paddling, and give you a chance to appreciate the inland scenery as well as the water. You'll even have the opportunity to soak your weary muscles in a hot spring. The combination of scenery, wildlife, and cozy cabins makes this a romantic getaway on every count. **More Information:** Misty Fjords National Monu-ment at 907-225-2148; www.fs.fed.us/r10/tongass.

If you and your partner are looking to spend some time alone in the wilderness, it's hard to find a better place for it than Wrangell-St. Elias National Park. America's largest national park covers over 20,000 square miles and is almost six times the size of Yellowstone. A couple of backpacking trails are relatively easy to reach. (Much of the park is only accessible by bush plane, so arranging trips can get a bit expensive.) From the small town of Chitina, you can arrange to be driven to the corner of McCarthy Road, the only road that leads into the park, and Kistina Road, which is a dirt side road. From there, you can hike up Kistina Road to either the Dixie Pass Trail or the Nugget Creek Trail. You'll be fording cold, Alaskan creeks, so be sure to bring a pair of warm, dry socks to change into when you make camp. If you hike along the Nugget Creek Trail to Dixie Pass, you can spend a couple of days exploring the area around the pass before hiking out again, for a total of three or four days. You're almost guaranteed to be completely alone in the wilderness. Just make sure you meet your arranged pickup at the road, or you could be waiting for quite a while for someone to come along and give you a ride. **More Information:** Wrangell-St. Elias National Park at 907-822-5234; www.nps.gov/wrst.

The 27-mile **Pinnell Mountain Trail**, 85 miles northeast of Fairbanks, offers you the unique opportunity to camp under the midnight sun. From June 18 to June 25, the sun doesn't set, and you can take fantastic pictures as it hovers over the horizon in the middle of the night. If that window of opportunity doesn't fit into your schedule, there are other great reasons to hike the trail. From late August onward, you'll be able to see the aurora borealis (northern lights) late in the night. If you've never seen this incredible phenomenon, you won't believe your

eyes. The sky is literally dancing above you in a colorful display. Is that romantic? The Japanese certainly think so. They consider it good luck to conceive a child under the aurora borealis, so if you run into a Japanese couple on the trail, make sure you make camp far enough away to give them a bit of privacy. Whether you're trying to breed or not, it's hard to imagine anything more magical than making love under the colorful, dancing sky. **More Information:** Pinnell Mountains National Recreation Trail at 907-454-2200; www.blm.gov/ak.

Hawaii

Most people think of a trip to Hawaii as a luxury vacation, where lounging on the beach is only interrupted by, oh, perhaps a bit of surfing. But there are some wonderful opportunities to experience Hawaii's natural beauty without staying at a five-star resort. Active volcanoes, lush forests, and dramatic coastlines make the islands a great place to explore by foot or by boat.

On the big island of Hawaii lies **Hawaii Volcanoes National Park.** Most people go for day walks in the park, enjoying the unique scenery. But if you're up for something a bit more rugged, you can try the tough climb up the Mauna Loa Summit Trail. At almost 14,000 feet, this is a major undertaking and altitude sickness is not uncommon, so don't take it lightly. But if you have some experience in the mountains, this will give you an opportunity to travel on a really different kind of terrain. The lava flows have turned the surface into something resembling the moon. Of course, the view from the top is unbeatable, and with so much effort needed to get there, you'll have a good chance of enjoying it by yourselves. **More Information:** Hawaii Volcanoes National Park at 808-985-6000; www.nps.gov/havo.

On Kauai, the must-see destination is the **Na Pali Coast.** The backpacking trail that follows the clifftops for 11 miles is challenging to say the least. Even experienced hikers find the dizzying heights and sometimes narrow ledges a bit daunting. But it's worth it. The views from

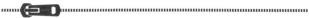

The Biggies: Glacier Bay National Park

Glacier Bay National Park has some outstanding scenery that is best enjoyed from the water. Unfortunately, it's a popular place, and the motorized tour boats can be rather daunting to the little kayaker.

One way to avoid the park's busiest areas is to paddle one of the bay's inlets. **Muir Inlet** can be paddled to the end and back in five or six days, and will give you views of a dozen glaciers. It's a remote paddle, but the million-dollar views are worth the extra effort to get there. Check with local tour operators to see who can provide transportation for you and your kayak to the mouth of the inlet. **More Information:** Glacier Bay National Park and Preserve at 907-697-2230; www.nps.gov/glba.

those cliff-top heights are undeniably beautiful, and the pounding surf below is inspiring. After a full day of hiking, you'll arrive at a gorgeous beach where you can camp for the night before making the return journey. If that sounds like more than you can handle, you can also explore the Na Pali Coast by sea kayak. Outfitters offer paddling trips where you're likely to see sea turtles, dolphins, seals, and tons of colorful sea birds while experiencing the towering cliffs and crashing surf from the water. **More Information:** Na Pali Coast State Park at 808-587-0300; www.hawaii.gov/dlnr/dsp.

On Maui, try visiting the **Haleakala National Park,** where you can hike in the Kipahulu Valley. Your hike will take you to scenic valleys, rainforest, and waterfalls, and dish out some fantastic ocean views. You'll also see shrines, temples, canoe ramps, and other evidence of Hawaiian habitation here many years ago. Most of the trails start from the ranger station. **More Information:** Haleakala National Park at 808-572-4400; www.nps.gov/hale.

Paddlers wanting to get off the beaten path can find their own little corner of paradise on the island of **Molokai.** The cliffs towering above you are some of the highest in the world. And down below, you'll have a chance to explore caves and paddle around tiny islands. One feature in particular is worth a visit: According to local legend, women who stay overnight at Molokai's fertile "Phallic Rock," or Kauleonanahoa, will go home pregnant. Camping on the island doesn't require any permits (except in the state and county parks), so you can pitch your tent wherever it looks good. That makes it even easier to find a corner of your very own and pretend it's your private tropical home. It doesn't get much more romantic than a private Hawaiian beach! **More Information:** Palaau State Park at 808-587-0300; www.hawaii.gov/dlnr/dsp.

Western Canada

Vancouver Island, off Canada's west coast, provides a natural playground for any kind of camper. Ferries from Vancouver make it easy to access, and the mountains

and coastline give you tons of exploring options. One popular pick for backpackers is the **West Coast Trail.** It offers 53 miles of sandy beaches, waterfalls, crashing shoreline, sandstone caves, and some of the world's tallest trees. Numbers are limited to 60 people per day, and they start from both ends of the trail. So while you won't be alone during the busy summer season, it shouldn't be ridiculously crowded. You'll be camping right on the beach, where you have a good chance of seeing dolphins, porpoises, orca, harbor seals, and sea lions. If you think a long walk on the beach is romantic, this may be the ideal trail for you.

Car campers also have some good choices both on Vancouver Island and the Gulf Islands between Vancouver Island and the mainland. The **Tofino** area is rated highly for car camping, with gorgeous scenery you can explore in dayhikes or in a kayak.

More ambitious paddlers can use Tofino as a base for paddling **Clayoquot Sound,** a UNESCO Biosphere Reserve. That means it's a protected ecosystem, internationally recognized for its unique biodiversity. This area is not for beginners, due to the challenging surf on many of the beaches, but it can make for several days of excellent paddling through uninhabited wilderness on the rugged Pacific Coast.

The less experienced should head to the **Broken Group Islands** in Pacific Rim Provincial Park, where you can paddle in a more sheltered area. The islands are south of Tofino, and the nearest town is Ucluelet. **More Information:** Vancouver Island Parks at 866-433-7272; www.bcparks.ca; or Pacific Rim National Park Reserve at 250-726-7721; www.pc.gc.ca/pn-np/bc/pacificrim.

When people claim a certain trail has "the most spectacular views in the Rockies," it's hard to resist. The **Skyline Trail** in Alberta's Jasper National Park is on the top of many must-do hike lists. At about 30 miles, it's usually a three-day trek, although some very energetic folks have been known to finish it in one long day. But why hurry through all of that wonderful scenery? The mountaintops and brilliant blue lakes beg you to stop and soak it all in. With just seven campsites, you'll need to reserve ahead, and you're likely to have company. But during the day, you'll have plenty of time and space to be on your own, marveling at nature's glory. **More Information:** Jasper National Park at 780-852-6176; www.pc.gc.ca/pn-np/ab/jasper.

The Biggies: Banff National Park

For some reason, no other part of the Canadian Rockies is as popular with tourists as Banff. It could be the quaint (or overpriced, depending on your perspective) skiing village right inside the park, or its proximity to a major city. Banff is just over an hour away from Calgary, Alberta, and it draws huge crowds all year. If you're up for a splurge, go ahead and book a couple of nights at the stunning Banff Springs Hotel and return from your dayhikes to a world of luxury.

Backpacking is also popular in Banff, but it may be worth dealing with the busy trails when the tradeoff is some of the most spectacular views in the Rockies. One classic trip is from Banff to **Mt. Assiniboine Provincial Park** in British Columbia, a distance of approximately 35 miles. Mt. Assiniboine is sometimes called the Matterhorn of the Rockies, and while climbing the mountain isn't an option for most of us, it's worth the trip just to enjoy the view from below.

Another good route (about 28 miles) starts at **Sunshine Meadows** ski area near Banff and goes over Ball Pass into British Columbia and down to the stunning **Floe Lake** in Kootenay National Park. The lake is named for the mini-icebergs that fall into it from surrounding glaciers. **More Information:** Banff National Park at 403-762-1550; www.pc.gc.ca/pn-np/ab/banff. Kootenay National Park at 250-347-9505; www.pc.gc.ca/pn-np/bc/kootenay. Mt. Assiniboine Provincial Park at 250-489-8540; www.env.gov.bc.ca/bcparks/explore/parkpgs/mt_assin.

If you think that visiting the Canadian Rockies during the summer means inevitably facing hordes of tourists, I've got a treat for you. **Willmore Wilderness Park** is at the northern end of the Rockies, where almost nobody goes. The reasons are twofold: First of all, it's about 200 miles from the nearest major city (Edmonton), and second, its mountains are not as tall as the more central sections of the Rockies, which draw bigger crowds. But if you want to leave to masses behind, there's no better place. You can choose from about 500 miles of trails and camp wherever you like, but the ridgelines are the best routes for backpackers because some of the lower trails see quite a bit of horse-trekking traffic, which makes them muddy. **More Information:** Willmore Wilderness Park at 780-865-8394; www.cd.gov.ab.ca/enjoying_alberta/parks.

Eastern Canada

Algonquin Provincial Park in central Ontario is legendary among paddlers. There are more than 1,300 miles of canoe routes to explore, making this a lifetime project for some Ontario residents. Even with its huge network of lakes and rivers, the best sites get booked out in the summer, so reserve ahead of your trip. The choicest spots will give you wonderful lakeside views and lots of privacy. It's very common to see moose in the park, but the bears and wolves are usually well hidden.

There are a number of campsites along the road that cuts through Algonquin's southern section, but they get very busy on summer weekends. If you're keen to do some car camping, make your way to the less-used campgrounds at the ends of dirt roads on the north and east sides of the park. Weekend warriors from Toronto rarely make the extra effort to get to these more remote places, so another hour or two of driving can give you a much better chance to enjoy a quiet night in the woods.

One of the best things about traveling up to central Ontario (or northern Maine) is that you can get a jump start on enjoying the romantic fall colors. This far north, the colors peak in late September and early October, so you can do an early fall trip up there, and then another one farther south later in the season. Cooler fall days also mean thinner crowds and fewer mosquitoes. Unless you're bug-proof, I'd suggest avoiding Algonquin during black fly season, from late May through June. They're surprisingly ferocious for their size and can make the whole trip miserable. **More Information:** Algonquin Provincial Park at 705-633-5572; www.ontarioparks.com.

Killarney Provincial Park in Ontario has one of those rare gems—a loop trail with spectacular scenery, lots of water sources, and isolated campsites. It's possible for very fit backpackers to do the 62-mile Lacloche Silhouette Trail in as little as five days, but seven to nine days is recommended. (It took me seven days, and I'm definitely no athlete!) Canoe enthusiasts can also enjoy the park by paddling a series of lakes with short portages linking them. Reservations are needed over the summer season, but because the interior sites are so spread out, you'll have as much privacy as you want at the end of the day. Most of the sites are on fabulous, scenic lakes. The park is famous for its shining white quartzite hills and pink granite, making it uniquely beautiful. If the loop trail is too long for you, don't worry. You can do part of the trail in either direction and backtrack out again, or you can just dayhike from the campground at the trailhead. **More Information:** Killarney Provincial Park at 705-287-2900; www.ontarioparks.com.

If you've been pining for the fjords, but you can't quite afford the flight to Norway, this is a good alternative. **The Saguenay Fjord** in Quebec is one of the biggest in the world, and it offers all of that spectacular landscape you'd expect from a fjord without the major airfare. Paddling the fjord is probably the best way to see it, so you can get up close and personal with the shoreline. For experienced sea kayakers, you'll be able to make the most of your independence if you follow the tide tables and remember that the water is very cold. The fjord is busiest in August, because that's when you've got a good chance of encountering beluga whales. So you'll have to decide whether paddling among these playful giants is worth the extra crowds, including motorized cruises.

You can also see the Saguenay from above by either car camping or backpacking. You'll get incredible views of the fjord below you and the dramatic cliffs rising on either side. There are plenty of villages along the length of the fjord, so you can grab supplies between destinations as you go. **More Information:** Saguenay St. Lawrence Marine Park at 418-235-4703; www.pc.gc.ca/amnc-nmca/qc/saguenay.

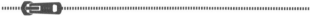

The Biggies:
Bay of Fundy

What makes the Bay of Fundy a biggie? The world's most extreme tides! The water level can vary by as much as 60 feet between high tide and low tide. The force of these tides (which can rush in fast enough to sweep you away if you're strolling along the water's edge) has carved out a dramatic landscape along the rocky shorelines. Like most biggies, the Bay of Fundy has been sadly over-commercialized. There are companies offering the chance to ride the tidal bore (a wave that pushes rivers the wrong way as the tide comes in), and even a simple walk around some of the more interesting rock formations now has an entrance fee.

The best way to experience Fundy's magic without feeling like you're in Disneyland is to visit **Fundy National Park** on the bay's north shore. You can explore the wilderness on land by staying at one of the three campgrounds in the park or the 13 backcountry tent sites. The bay itself is best explored on day trips, since you'll have to be well aware of the tides and conditions. For longer shoreline trips, experienced paddlers can study the tide tables and be prepared for cold water, or play it safe and take a guided trip. **More Information:** Fundy National Park at 506-887-6000; www.pc.gc.ca/pn-np/nb/fundy.

Appendix 2:

The World as
YOUR
OUTDOOR
BEDROOM

Getting farther away from home to explore parks around the world allows you to experience a wider variety of landscapes and climates. You'll have an opportunity to see different wildlife and flora and experience firsthand places that you've read about in adventure tales or seen in movies. World travel can be pricey, but you can knock the costs down a few notches by traveling in the wilderness and staying in a tent. The trip of a lifetime doesn't have to include expensive hotels and resorts to be the most romantic thing you've ever done together.

An international camping trip can be luxurious, staying in mountain chalets and having some of your gear transported for you while you hike to the next chalet. Or it can be incredibly remote and adventurous, exploring jungles or deserts where few tourists dare to venture.

This section doesn't focus on staying away from the crowds, because if you're going to travel all the way to another continent to camp, I figure you should see the best of the best, no matter how many other people are there. Everyone has slightly different priorities when it comes to what they want to see, and specialty publishers like Lonely Planet and Trailblazer have excellent guidebooks to help you sift through all of the other choices available. We'll be taking a look at a few global highlights here, but if you're going to be in the country anyway, you might want to see more while you're there, and exploring outside is a great way to get a real flavor for a country.

Mexico and South America

If you're a fan of beach camping, head to **Baja California** in Mexico. This skinny peninsula is lined with beaches on both sides just waiting for you and your tent. If you've got a four-wheel-drive vehicle, you can get onto the back roads and find completely deserted stretches of beach that go for miles. So stock up with some food and water and do a bit of tropical car camping. **More Information:** Mexico Tourism at 888-401-3880 (US toll free); www.visitmexico.com.

The **Galapagos Islands:** It's hard to resist the lure of this remote cluster of islands that inspired Charles Darwin

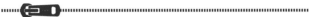

Make Mexico Extra Hot!

Mexicans make hot chocolate with combinations of spices, including hot chilies. Take some of their specialty with you on your Mexican camping adventures and it will definitely get your libido going full tilt.

with their unique wildlife. The Galapagos are a world treasure, and therefore they are very heavily protected. If you want to visit, you'll have to go with one of the tour companies permitted to organize trips there. Different trips focus on different activities, so if you're a paddler, make sure you take a tour that includes kayaking around the shorelines. You'll be able to get very close to the animals and see some unique species. Most trips also include snorkeling and/or scuba diving so you can check out the local sea life. A trip like this is a once-in-a-lifetime opportunity, so it's worth sacrificing your dedication to independent travel for a chance to see wildlife that just doesn't exist anywhere else in the world. To share an experience that so few will ever have is a real gift to your relationship. **More Information:** Galapagos National Park at www.galapagos.org or www.galapagospark.org.

The **Amazon Rainforest** lives in our collective imagination as one of the most remote and primitive places left on Earth. Giant snakes, jungle cats, and piranhas make their home alongside tribal cultures that have managed to continue living in their traditional ways, out of reach of the modern world. This vast region spans from Brazil in the east to Ecuador and Chile in the west and Bolivia in the south. A visit to the Amazon feels more like an expedition than a holiday, but it's an adventure you're not likely to forget. So if the two of you have a bit of explorer in you, this could be your dream destination. It's nature at its most raw, and there's no doubt that you'll just be a humble guest in its presence.

Most people opt for a guided tour through the jungle or down a river. For those who choose to go it alone, you will probably still need some help getting to your destination. Locals can take you to the starting point of your journey in a motorized canoe and arrange to pick you up at another designated point. If you're going to attempt an independent river trip or rainforest trek, make sure you are well-supplied and prepared. **More Information:** Ecuador Ministry of Tourism at www.vivecuador.com/html2/eng/home.htm, Chile Tourism Promotion Corporation at www.visit-chile.org, Brazil Tourism Office at www.braziltourism.org, or Bolivia Vice-Ministry of Tourism at www.turismobolivia.bo/index_en.php.

The **Andes** have some of the most spectacular mountains you could ever hope to see. Running almost the entire length of South America, your options for visiting the Andes are too many to name. Scaling the peaks is beyond the reach of most mortals, but admiring them from close up is just a matter of packing our bags and heading south. **More Information:** Chile Tourism Promotion Corporation at www.visit-chile.org. **Further Reading:** *Trekking in the Patagonian Andes* (Lonely Planet).

In Chile, a visit to **Torres del Paine National Park** will give you a taste of unforgettable Patagonian landscapes. There are a number of trekking options here, but the classic route is the Torres del Paine Circuit. It takes anywhere from a week to 10 days to complete the circuit, and while there are refugios (hiking huts) to stay in, they are not very well-maintained, and they're crowded during busy times. Bringing a tent gives you the option of having your nights to yourselves. The trek goes through forests, rocky gullies, streams, and bogs, showing off outstanding scenery along the way—huge spires, hanging glaciers, giant granite walls, and stunning lakes. If your time is limited, you can do a shorter, three-day trek that's usually called the "W." **More Information:** Chile Tourism Promotion Corporation at www.visit-chile.org. **Further Reading:** *Trekking in the Patagonian Andes* (Lonely Planet).

While Patagonia is very heavily visited, there are still more remote areas if you hate to be surrounded by other

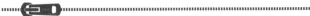

Go for
The Gold

The Incan empire once covered almost the entire west coast of South America. They built elaborate cities and roads, and created detailed statues covered in gold and silver. Unfortunately, the conquering Spanish armies melted down most of their treasures, so all that's left to admire is the stonework. However, there are still many treasures, albeit of the smaller variety, to be seen (and purchased) in the Andes.

Why not use your trip to the Andes to put a little sparkle back into this ancient area, and your relationship? At a key moment in your trip (visiting a ruined city, or at the top of a wonderful vista), surprise your partner with a gift of gold or silver. Anything from earrings to a necklace or even a tie pin is light and easy to store away in your trekking gear. Just one warning to the men: Rings are only advisable if you're actually going to pop the question. An unexpected gift will definitely light up your partner's eyes after a long day of mountain trekking.

trekkers. In Argentina, **Perito Moreno National Park** is only accessible by dirt road. This park is slowly being developed, so you'll be able to find campgrounds and hiking trails where only a few years ago there was nothing but wilderness. Because there are so few visitors to this park, you'll have a chance to see more wildlife, and, of course, you'll be able to enjoy your time together without any (human) onlookers. **More Information:** Argentina Secretariat of Tourism at www.turismo.gov.ar/eng/menu.htm, or Argentina National Parks at www.parquesnacionales.gov.ar.

If you're interested in South America's history, you'll be tempted to take a trip along the Inca Trail. But due to overuse, the government has made it illegal to hike the trail unless you're on an organized tour, so as far as solitude goes, you're out of luck. But if you're not dead set on getting to Machu Picchu, why not get away from the steady stream of walkers and explore some of the other Incan archeological sites? **Choquequirao** is one of those sites. Sitting on a high ridge more than 5000 feet above the Apurimac River, this "lost city" of the Incas lacks the constant flood of tours of Machu Picchu. The surrounding mountains are just as spectacular as the city itself, so there are many rewards for making the journey. The construction of a footbridge over the Apurimac River makes the site much more accessible than it once was, so if you're up for a bit of a trek, you can discover this ancient place before the tour companies do. **More Information:** Commission for the Promotion of Peru at www.peru.info/perueng.asp, or the Peruvian Embassy at www.peruvianembassy.us/visiting-peru-destination-guide-choquequirao.php.

Europe

The Alps have been the playground of the Europeans for centuries. They've been hiking, climbing, and exploring these mountains for so long, the Alps have become one of the most developed trekking destinations in the world. A hiking trip in the Alps can be as luxurious or as challenging as you like. If you're going to Europe for an adventure holiday, I suggest avoiding the month of August, when all of the locals take their holidays.

The highest peak of the Alps is also the focus of its most famous hike, the **Tour de Mont Blanc** or **TMB**. This 120-mile route around Mont Blanc usually takes about 11 days to complete, giving you breathtaking views from every angle. Because of the trail's location, you'll actually pass through three different countries to complete it: France, Italy, and Switzerland. Of course popularity has its price, and the *refuges* (huts) are likely to fill up over the summer. But you can't get much more civilized than ending your day's hike with a cozy bed and a well-cooked meal. **More Information:** French Tourist Office at www.francetourism.com, Swiss National Tourist Office at www.myswitzerland.com/en.cfm/home, or Italian Tourism Board at www.italiantourism.com. **Further Reading:** *Tour*

of Mont Blanc: Complete Trekking Guide (Cicerone), or *Walking in the Alps* (Lonely Planet).

Another popular route is the Alps is the 110-mile Walker's Haute Route from Chamonix, France, to Zermatt, Switzerland. The great thing about this route is that you can cheat if you want to! The whole thing takes about two weeks, but because of the great system of public transport, you can skip some of the stages by taking a bus to the next access point. The trail has views of two of the most famous mountains in the Alps, Mont Blanc in France and the Matterhorn in Switzerland. Again, you can stay in refuges or village inns if you want to be pampered, or go to the campgrounds in the valleys if you'd prefer to have a more traditional camping trip. Maybe a combination of both would be ideal? **More Information:** Chamonix Tourist Office at www.chamonix.net/english/trek/haute_route_walk, French Tourist Office at www.francetourism.com, or Swiss National Tourist Office at www.myswitzerland.com/en.cfm/home. **Further Reading:** *Walking in the Alps* (Lonely Planet), or *Chamonix to Zermatt: A Walker's Haute Route* (Cicerone).

If the Alps are a little too developed for your liking, you might prefer to head to the Pyrenees. This mountain range stretches along the entire border between France and Spain, and you can walk 300 miles or more across the whole thing. The **Haute Randonnée Pyrenéenne (HRP)** is a famous route that follows the ridgeline and crosses between France and Spain numerous times. It's only recommended for people who are experienced in mountain conditions because you'll be on an exposed ridge most of the time, but no technical climbing skills are required. If you want to do the whole thing, it's a big commitment. Six weeks or more may be needed to get across. But most people do a section of the route instead, enjoying the phenomenal views.

The Pyrenees also offer two lower routes from one end to the other, the 600 plus-mile **GR10** in France and the 520-mile **GR11** in Spain. Ironically, these walks are both tougher than the HRP because they have more ups and downs, while the ridge route stays high for the entire time. The GR10 is the older and more developed of the routes, where it is possible to trek without a tent or much food and rely on refuges. On the Spanish side, things are not as developed, so you'll need to camp and be more self-sufficient. **More Information:** French Tourist Office at www.francetourism.com, Spain Tourism Office at www.spain.info, Pyrenees National Park at www.parc-pyrenees.com, or the Pyrenees Guide (an unofficial but informative website) at www.pyreneesguide.com. **Further Reading on the HRP:** *The Pyrenean Haute Route* (Cicerone), or *Trekking in the Pyrenees* (Trailblazer). **Further Reading on the GR10 and GR11:** *The GR10 Trail* (Cicerone), or *Through the Spanish Pyrenees GR11* (Cicerone).

The British have always been big on walking for recreation. Having a large population living for centuries on a relatively small island means that there are not many vast wilderness areas remaining, yet there are still lots of opportunities to have an adventure on foot. Rather than trying to escape the history of human presence in Britain, embrace it with a journey along a piece of history itself. **Hadrian's Wall** was built during the golden age of the Roman Empire, with construction starting in 122 AD, to separate Roman Britain from the "barbarians" in what is now Scotland. A cycleway (opened in 2006) follows a 173-mile route from coast to coast. You can follow any portion of the route, staying in campgrounds or local villages overnight. Walkers can also follow the 84-mile **Hadrian's Wall Path** through rolling fields and rugged moors. **More Information:** Northumberland National Park Authority at www.nationaltrail.co.uk/hadrianswall. **Further Reading:** *Hadrian's Wall Path* (Trailblazer).

For traditionalists, there's only one way to walk England all the way across, and it takes about two weeks. The popular Coast-to-Coast Walk goes from St. Bees Head (Whitehaven) to Robin Hood's Bay (near Whitby) and is about 190 miles long. It's not exactly wilderness all of the way, but you will walk through three national parks and experience a variety of terrain that includes mountains, moors, and lowlands. Since you'll pass through a number of villages on your journey, you only have to carry food for a few days at a time, making this one of the most doable long-distance hikes you're likely to find anywhere. **More Information:** Whitehaven Tourist Information Centre at www.coast2coast.co.uk. **Further Reading:** *Coast-to-Coast Path* (Trailblazer), or *Walking in Britain* (Lonely Planet).

Of course the Scottish believe they are the only *real* walkers in Britain. They've been roaming the highlands for centuries, and the rugged beauty of that scenery is much more wild than anything you'll find in England. To experience some of Scotland's most famous landscape, try trekking the **Great Glen**. It's a four-day, 70-mile route that takes you along the length of Loch Ness, where you can keep an eye out for monsters. You'll also get some wonderful mountain scenery along the way, and pass a few ruined castles. This route from Inverness to Fort William can be hiked at any time of year, but it can be icy in the winter. **More Information:** www.greatglenway.fsnet.co.uk. **Further Reading:** *Walking in Scotland* (Lonely Planet).

If you want to really experience the wild side of Scotland, head for the **Cairngorms National Park**. This area is almost exactly in the middle of Scotland. There are many hiking options in the park, including some overnight routes that take you up to wonderful viewpoints in the mountains. **More Information:** Cairngorms National Park Authority at www.cairngorms.co.uk. **Further Reading:** *Walking in Scotland* (Lonely Planet).

If you like your adventures on the cold side, make some time to explore Scandinavia. Sweden, Finland, Denmark, and Norway have been drawing people into their spectacular outdoors for generations. Norway's fjords are, of course, legendary. Less famous (as least internationally) are their mountains. Jotunheimen means "home of the giants," and that's where Norwegians go to trek among the mountains, glaciers, snowy peaks, and bright, blue lakes. Jotunheimen National Park offers all kinds of experiences for the hardy camper. You can stay at full-service lodges with beds and hot food, simpler self-service lodges, or "unserviced" huts, where you'll be on your own for food, but you will also be, well, on your own! You can pitch a tent instead if that's more your style. The park features a weblike network of trails, so even during the most popular times (weekends in July and August), you can plan your trip to be as friendly or as remote as you like. **More Information:** Norway Directorate for Nature Management at www.sognefjord.no.

Asia

Nepal is a mecca for mountain enthusiasts. The thought of even catching a glimpse of Mt. Everest draws thousands of people to this remote corner of the world. Climbing Everest is challenging, risky, and ridiculously expensive, but many more of us can bask in its glory by taking a trek to **Everest Base Camp**. Even this humble location is high in the Himalayas, and you'll have to acclimatize several times during your trek to avoid altitude sickness at the 18,370-foot base camp. The walk is only recommended from October to May. **More Information:** Nepal Tourism at www.tourism.gov.np/trekkingagenciaslists or the VisitNepal at www.visitnepal.com/trekking. **Further Reading:** *Trekking in the Nepal Himalaya* (Lonely Planet) or *Trekking in the Everest Region* (Trailblazer).

If that sounds a little too cold or too high for your tastes, how about a tropical getaway in southern Thailand? **Khao**

Listen to the Singing Lake

If you're going on a trek to Everest Base Camp, it's easy to get tunnel vision and focus on your goal without enjoying the journey. Try taking a side trip to **Gokyo Lake**, where the constant freezing and thawing cycle of the lake can make it sound like whales singing.

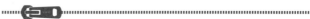

Thai Beach Life

After exploring the rainforest of southern Thailand, take a couple extra days to enjoy its famous beaches. If you're all adventured out, you can simply lounge on the white sand and cool off in the turquoise waters. Or if you're up for more action, try paddling along the coast in a canoe, either on your own or with an organized tour. **Krabi** is a great starting point for hitting the water, and it's just a short journey southwest from Khao Sok. Yes, the island resort of Phuket is closer, but it's more touristy and expensive, too. So head farther south, find a bit of beach to call your own and bask in Thailand's natural beauty. **More information:** Tourism Authority of Thailand: www.tourismthailand.org.

Sok National Park is a popular place to explore. Too popular, some would say, as tourists from nearby Phuket come for a lazy visit on their day away from the beach. But for the more adventurous visitors, Khao Sok has a lot to offer. This dense, lush rainforest provides a home for wild elephants, leopards, sun bears, and even a few tigers. You may never get a chance to spot these elusive residents, but the farther you stray from the lodges and facilities, the better your odds. If you feel uneasy exploring on your own, there are plenty of guided treks available. If you do head off on the trails unsupervised, keep an eye on your legs, as leeches are abundant. Most visitors stay in treehouse bungalows, which provide a fun, unique way to enjoy the rainforest. Now you're really going to get a chance to bring that Tarzan fantasy to life! **More Information:** National Parks, Wildlife, and Conservation Department of Thailand at www.dnp.go.th/index_eng.asp, or the Tourism Authority of Thailand at www.tourismthailand.org.

If you're looking for something more remote, it's hard to imagine any place that would fit the bill better than northeastern Cambodia, in the province of Ratanakiri. *Apocalypse Now* was set here, but you're not likely to find any renegade colonel on your trip. **Virachay National Park** is a wild rainforest that you can explore from the back of an elephant, or, for the real *Apocalypse Now* experience, by boat. You definitely won't run into any crowds of tourists in this remote corner of Southeast Asia. Cambodia is only just beginning to create a tourist infrastructure after decades of war and suffering. They are starting to discover that they have something to offer the world, and you can be one of the first to take them up on their offer. **More Information:** Cambodia Ministry of Tourism at www.mot.gov.kh/attraction_park.asp.

Paddlers may not have thought to put Japan on their list of places to visit, but if you leave behind the urban madness of Tokyo, you'll get to see the country's more peaceful side. The **Noto Peninsula,** in the center of the north coast, is shaped like a bent finger and offers 360 miles of picturesque coastline for determined paddlers. The eastern side is quite touristy and developed, but it is also more sheltered and easier to paddle. Once you round the peninsula to the north, the more exposed waters make this section a trip for experienced sea kayakers only. The mountains inland provide a stunning backdrop for your journey, and the inlets, eroded rock formations, hot springs, and rice fields keep it interesting closer to sea level. **More Information:** Japan Tourism Bureau at www.jnto.go.jp/eng.

Africa

When you think about a camping trip to Africa, the word "safari" immediately comes to mind. The idea of seeing lions, cheetahs, giraffes, zebras, and rhinos in their natural habitat is hard to beat. African safaris come in all shapes and sizes. The most popular areas for visiting wildlife reserves are in the savannahs of **Kenya** and **Tanzania,** and also in eastern **South Africa.** Camping safaris

give you the feeling of sleeping among the wild animals, but with armed guides on standby just in case they get a little too curious! You'll get what you pay for, so if you're happy with uninspired food and basic tents, you can save some cash. If you want to splurge, you can find anything from huge, canvas tents with ensuite washrooms, to five-star hunting lodges. But the accommodations are not the point. You want to see Africa's wild beasts, so make sure you're up early to catch them at their most active. If you'd rather not get stuck with a guided trip, it's possible to rent a four-by-four and do your own safari. **More Information:** Tanzania Tourist Board at www.tanzaniatouristboard.com, or Kenya Tourist Board at www.magicalkenya.com. **Further Reading:** *Watching Wildlife: Eastern Africa* (Lonely Planet), or *Watching Wildlife: Southern Africa* (Lonely Planet).

Apart from going on safari, the most popular adventure in Tanzania is climbing **Mt. Kilimanjaro,** which, at 19,340 feet, is the highest mountain in Africa. "Kili" is a nontechnical climb, so anyone in good shape can do it. Most companies offer a guided, four-day ascent and return. If you want to be a little different, do a traverse instead. This will make the journey a day or two longer, but at least for the descent you will lose the crowds. Kilimanjaro is the tallest freestanding volcano in the world, so you can look forward to incredible views and a great feeling of accomplishment when you set foot on the summit. **More Information:** Tanzania National Parks at www.tanzaniaparks.com, or Tanzania Tourist Board at www.tanzaniatouristboard.com. **Further Reading:** *Kilimanjaro: A Trekking Guide to Africa's Highest Mountain* (Trailblazer).

If you're up for a ramble in South Africa, you can visit the **Northern Drakensberg** and choose how far and how challenging you'd like your adventure to be. One popular route takes you from an area called the Amphitheatre in Royal Natal National Park, to Cathedral in the Mlambonja Wilderness Area. The Amphitheatre's sheer basalt cliffs are more than 3,000 feet tall, and surround you for their

2.5-mile width. It's a dramatic start to four or five days of raw African mountain scenery. The sharp pinnacles of rock seem to pierce the sky, and the amount of climbing along this route means that it's best tackled in spring or fall when the heat is less extreme. Cathedral Peaks at the end of the trek features four peaks over 10,000 feet high. Add another day at the end of your trip to climb one, if you've still got the energy.

More hardcore adventurers can do a traverse of the **Drakensberg Mountains.** You're looking at 10 to 12 days of backpacking over high passes (around 10,000 feet), so this is for people who like a challenge. The less ambitious can camp in any of the national parks in the Drakensberg Mountains and take dayhikes to explore the area. **More Information:** Drakensberg Tourism at www.drakensberg-tourism.com.

At the opposite end of Africa, Morocco holds its own appeal. The ancient cultures in this area are still alive and well, and they'll make your trekking experience all the more exotic. You can take on North Africa's highest mountain, Mt. Toubkal, as part of the **Toubkal Circuit.** Tour companies organize trips from Marrakech, and use mules to transport a lot of the supplies to unburden

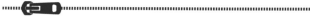

Good Things Come to Those Who Hike

Your trek through the Drakensberg to Cathedral finishes at the doorstep of the Cathedral Peak Hotel. Why not book ahead and treat yourselves to a luxurious night to cap off your journey?

Use the hotel's steam bath to ease your tired muscles, have a gourmet meal in their dining room, and enjoy the luxury of a comfortable bed. There's even a beauty therapist available in case you want to return from your trek with a perfect pedicure!

the travelers. You'll be thankful for that when you start ascending the 12,000-foot mountain. Along the way, you'll pass traditional cliffside Berber villages, where life is relatively unchanged from centuries ago. You'll be staying in local villages, and getting to see the Berber way of life. Of course, there's a great view from the summit, with the fertile fields back toward Marrakech, and the beginnings of the Sahara heading south. The whole trip usually lasts eight days, and is a side of Africa that few foreigners ever see. **More Information:** Moroccan National Tourist Office at www.visitmorocco.org. **Further Reading:** *Trekking in the Moroccan Atlas* (Trailblazer).

Australia and New Zealand

A trip Down Under can give you just about any kind of adventure you could imagine. In Australia and New Zealand, you can visit rocky deserts, tropical rainforests, snow-capped mountains, active volcanoes, glaciers, fjords, and great beaches.

Australia is roughly the same size as the continental US, but with a population of only around 20 million people. So if you thought there were some big wilderness areas left in the US, just imagine a country the same size with less than 10 percent of the people! The wildlife here is unlike any in other parts of the world, from kangaroos to koalas, to the impossible-looking platypus.

One of the most popular and unique places in Australia is **Fraser Island,** off the east coast. This is the world's biggest sand island, but it's more than just a great beach. There is a whole rainforest growing out of the dunes. The sand is such a great filter that the creeks running out of Fraser Island have the clearest water you're ever likely to see. Most people explore the island during a three-day, self-driving tour in a four-by-four. But if you want to have a more peaceful encounter, you can hike to the most impressive sights instead. A four-day loop will take you to dense forests, gorgeous lakes, and miles of beach. If you're going to swim, I recommend the lakes and rivers. The coast of Fraser Island is a favorite hangout for sharks. **More Information:** Queensland Parks and Wildlife

Service at www.epa.qld.gov.au, or Tourism Australia at www.australia.com. **Further Reading:** *Walking in Australia* (Lonely Planet).

If you're up for a long trail, try the **Great South West Walk** along Australia's south coast. The walk's location between the major cities of Melbourne and Adelaide makes it easy to access. The whole 155 miles takes about two weeks to complete, although there's a town about halfway along if you want to do a shorter trip. Your spectacular coastal scenery will be interrupted only by the track heading through eucalyptus forests and rainforests. **More Information:** Portland Visitor Information Center at www.greatsouthwestwalk.com. **Further Reading:** *Walking in Australia* (Lonely Planet).

The lure of the outback is hard to resist. The bright red rocks positively glow in the early-morning and late-evening light. The vast nothingness of it all is overwhelming yet peaceful. Most visitors head for the iconic Ayers Rock, and while it's definitely worth a look, there's much more to the outback than one gigantic monolith. The **Larapinta Trail** starts from Alice Springs (the outback's biggest town) and goes west for almost 150 miles in 12 sections. Each section is accessible by road, so if you don't want to do the whole thing (a 20-day journey), you can leave a car at the next trailhead. **More Information:** Northern Territory Parks & Wildlife Service at www.nt.gov.au/nreta/parks. **Further Reading:** *Walking in Australia* (Lonely Planet).

For the serious trekker, no trip to Australia would be complete without visiting Tasmania. The hiking in Tassie is the best in the country, and there are far fewer people there than in any of the other non-desert areas. The **Overland Track** is Tasmania's big walk, perhaps the premiere multiday walk in Australia. The alpine moors, rainforest, and rugged peaks will make you forget about the beaches and deserts of mainland Australia. It takes five to seven days to cover the 50 miles of track, and you can stay in either huts or tents. This route does get pretty popular over the summer, and bookings are required from November

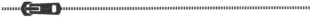

Getting into the Swag of Things

Traditionally, the cowboys of the Aussie outback have used a "swag" when sleeping outside. It's basically a canvas bag with a thin mattress inside, carried as a bed roll. You can throw your sleeping bag in there and make a very comfy bed, even on top of rock.

If you're camping in the desert, do it like the Aussies and forget the tent. (Assuming there's no rain in the forecast, of course.) By bedding down in swags under the desert sky, you'll be in for some of the most spectacular stargazing you'll find anywhere. The sky seems to go on forever in every direction, and there are no cities nearby to dilute the darkness. Sleeping uncovered is incredibly liberating, and making love under the stars will make your stay in the outback unforgettable.

through April, but the cooler weather in spring and fall will give you more space to yourselves. **More Information:** Cradle Mountain Visitor Center at www.parks.tas.gov.au. **Further Reading:** *Walking in Australia* (Lonely Planet).

If you're looking for car camping or shorter backpacking opportunities, you'd do well to visit the **Flinders Ranges** in South Australia. There are tons of dayhikes in the mountains, many of them within anyone's skill level. The overnight loop around **Wilpena Pound** is a local favorite, giving you a chance to admire this big, bowl-shaped feature from every angle. **More Information:** South Australia Parks & Wildlife Service at www.parks.sa.gov.au. **Further Reading:** *Walking in Australia* (Lonely Planet).

New Zealand is much smaller than Australia—about the same size as Britain (without Northern Ireland)—but no less of a camper's dream. About one third of the country has been set aside as protected wilderness. Backpacking, or "tramping" as they call it, is a national obsession, so there are trails everywhere. The Department of Conservation maintains more than 1000 backcountry huts all over the country. Paddlers can enjoy everything from silent lakes to raging rivers and some of the best costal scenery in the world.

New Zealand's popularity with backpackers has in a sense been its downfall. The government decided to label the 10 most popular routes in the country as the "great walks," and they've done such a great job marketing them that some are now booked to capacity months in advance. The best way to experience New Zealand's great variety of backcountry is to skip the great walks and hike on other nearby tracks. The scenery will be just as stunning, but the crowds will be much thinner and the huts less packed.

Fiordland National Park contains the most famous hike in New Zealand, the Milford Track. Unless you feel like booking six months in advance, I suggest you skip it and do one of the other excellent trails in the park. For any easy route try the five-day **Hollyford Track**, which stays at a low elevation the whole way. The moderately challenging **Routeburn** and **Kepler** tracks are both "great walks," but they're not as crowded as the Milford Track, so you should be able to walk them as long is you're not visiting over Christmas, when all of the locals will be off work. The three-day **Tuatapere Hump Ridge Track** offers great views for backpackers on a tighter schedule.

If you want isolation in Fiordland, your best bet is the remote **Dusky Track**. It's a tougher route than most of the other Fiordland trails, and harder to get to, so very few people bother with it. There are steep climbs and several walkwires to use for river crossings. This is New Zealand at its most rugged, so if you're up for the challenge, you'll really be able to appreciate the wilderness. Any trip to Fiordland is likely to involve some rain, so be prepared for wet conditions at any time of year.

Backpacking in New Zealand's Southern Alps can be a real challenge, with high passes and sudden changes in the weather. One of the best places to explore the alpine scenery is **Nelson Lakes National Park.** This northern part of the range is a bit more sheltered than the areas farther south, and so the weather there tends to be drier and less extreme. There are a number of well-marked routes as well, which can be hard to find in other parts of the mountains where local trampers simply follow the ridges and valleys. The **Travers Valley** is one of the most accessible parts of the park, and has a good network of trails and huts to choose from. It's all fairly challenging because of the alpine passes, but it's also well-used and well-marked. As you may have guessed by the park's name, there are some wonderful alpine lakes in the area where paddlers can soak in the scenery and even do some fishing. For car campers, day walks are plentiful and there are several campgrounds, although most have only basic facilities like toilets and water.

The North Island of New Zealand is where you'll find all of the geothermal action. Volcanoes, geysers, and sulfur pools fill the center of the island. The most popular day walk in the country, the **Tongariro Crossing**, is a full day of stunning volcanic terrain including brilliantly colored lakes and steaming vents. It's busy all summer, and weekends in spring and fall, but it might just be worth dealing with the crowds. To get a better feel for the area, and some more varied terrain, you can do the four-day **Tongariro Northern Circuit**, which circles the cone-shaped peak of Mt. Ngauruhoe. It includes most of the Crossing day walk as part of the route. It's a "great walk" though, so it could be crowded during peak times.

A more solitary option would be the **Mt. Ruapehu Round-the-Mountain Track**. It takes most people five or six days and circles the largest of the three volcanic peaks in Tongariro National Park. You can then do the Tongariro Crossing as a dayhike before or after the circuit and see all of the main scenery without the constant stream of hikers and crowded huts. More Information: New Zealand Department of Conservation at www.doc.govt.nz. **Further Reading:** *Tramping in New Zealand* (Lonely Planet) or *101 Great Tramps in New Zealand* (Reed).

Absolutely Everything
You Need to
GET OUTSIDE
AND GET IT ON

Books, Toys, and More for Wild Couples

Good Vibrations: www.goodvibes.com. San Francisco's favorite sex shop is online, providing a wealth of information and products, including a wide variety of high-quality toys and a great selection of books and videos.

D.Vice Designer Sex Gear: www.dvice.co.nz. If you're Down Under and looking for quality sex toys that have been put through their paces, check out New Zealand's d.vice. In case you can't go for a visit, check out their website, which has a comprehensive advice section to help you find the right products and use them the right way.

Talk Sex with Sue: www.talksexwithsue.com. Sue Johanson has been dishing out sex advice on radio and TV for more than 30 years, so she knows a thing or two! Her website has helpful information on a whole range of topics. She also sells selected products through the site, including her own books, *Talk Sex, Sex is Perfectly Natural But Not Naturally Perfect,* and *Sex, Sex, and More Sex* (all from Penguin).

Mating in Captivity: Reconciling the Erotic + the Domestic by Esther Perel (HarperCollins 2006). Perel's intriguing book about how hard it can be to have great sex in a long-term relationship raised a few eyebrows with some unconventional advice. If the status quo isn't working for you, check out Perel's ideas on how to turn up the heat when the sparks have stopped.

Cosmo's Aqua Kama Sutra by the editors of *Cosmopolitan* (Hearst Books 2006). If you're turned on by the idea of sex in the water, here's an entire book of positions to try. The best thing about it is the book is waterproof, so you can take it with you for easy reference.

The Wild Guide to Sex and Loving by Siobhan Kelly (Amorata Press 2002). This book covers everything from sensual massage to S&M in full color. If you're looking for new ideas to spice things up, this could be a place to start. There is text, but in this case, a picture is worth a thousand words or more.

Superhotsex by Tracey Cox (DK Adult 2006). This book is aimed at long-term couples trying to stoke the fires of passion. It even has some suggestions for getting it on outdoors. If you're in need of some fresh ideas, this is an inspiring read.

Singles Outdoor Resources

Fitness Singles: www.fitness-singles.com. Looking for someone who shares your passion for the outdoors so you can become a wild couple? Check out this dating website and click on your activity of choice. They've got everything from adventure racing to horseshoes, so you're bound to find someone who likes the same activities as you.

Date Active: www.dateactive.co.uk. This British website is for meeting people into outdoor activities. Hook up with others in your area who can take your love life into the wilderness.

Meet Market Adventures: www.meetmarketadventures.com. This isn't a dating service. Instead, they run events where groups of single people who enjoy the same activities can meet, and maybe hook up. This expanding company now schedules events in New York, Philadelphia, Chicago, Toronto, Ottawa, Montreal, Calgary, and Vancouver.

Events and Adventures: www.eventsandadventures.com. Similar to Meet Market Adventures, this company sets up events for singles who like to get active. They have locations in Seattle, Houston, Dallas, and Minneapolis, and they also have a partner company that plans events in Orlando, Tampa, South Florida, and Atlanta (www.eventsandadventuresfl.com).

Mosaic Outdoors Clubs: Jewish singles looking for an outdoorsy match can check out the activities at the Mosaic clubs in 21 American cities, and in Toronto. Their main website is www.mosaicoutdoor.org.

Gay and Lesbian Outdoor Resources

Gay Outdoors: www.gayoutdoors.org. This site is just for the boys. It features a variety of outdoor sports but has a section devoted to camping and hiking. You'll find articles, events, discussion groups, and even online dating. There's also information on nude campgrounds.

IGLOO, the International Gay and Lesbian Outdoors Organization: www.radix.net/~erewhon/igloo/igloo.html. These guys win the best acronym award! This site provides contact information for local gay and lesbian outdoors groups all over the US and Canada, as well as several other countries. If you're not sure where to look for like-minded campers in your state, this is a good place to start.

Camping

GORP: www.gorp.com. This website has all kinds of great information on places to go, both in the US and around the world. There are trip reports for backpacking, paddling, and international vacations, plus articles on a variety of topics. It also has gear guides, packing lists, and park information.

Great Outdoors: www.greatoutdoors.com. This site has two sides, one for online gear and clothing shopping, and the other for full-length articles. The articles make for some good inspiration if you're looking for new ideas.

Outdoor Adventure Canada: www.outdooradventurecanada.com. Look here for articles, reviews, and tips for backpackers, car campers, and paddlers. The focus is on Canada, but the information is mostly universal. The discussion forums are great places to pick people's minds and get firsthand tips on trips.

The Camping Guide: www.thecampingguide.com. Features articles and retail links for camping, hunting, and other outdoor gear. You'll also find articles about some interesting destinations.

Safe Trip Canada: www.safetrip.ca. This is for trips in Canada only. Simply register your trip plan or float plan online, along with your contact details. If you don't report back when you are due to return from your trip, the people who run the site will try to contact you using the details you supplied. If they are unable to contact you after an hour of trying, they will call the police in the area where your trip is taking place and report you missing, passing on your trip plan details. This is great for people who don't have a reliable friend or family member to check up on them.

Outside Magazine: In print or online at outside.away.com. *Outside* is one of the best-known outdoor magazines around. It covers a wide range of topics, including camping, backpacking, skiing, paddling, cycling, climbing, running, and more. You'll find inspiring articles, gear reviews, book reviews, and ideas to incorporate into your future trips.

Outpost Magazine: In print or online at www.outpost-magazine.com. This Canadian outdoor magazine has great articles on camping and adventure travel, plus health and more.

How to Shit in the Woods by Kathleen Meyer (Ten Speed Press 1989). It has become a camping classic—the book about what we all need to know, but don't want to admit we don't know! A second edition with an additional chapter was released in 1994, so if your copy is older, you could be missing the latest "poop."

Backpacking

Trails.com: www.trails.com. Trail reports and even topographic maps can be found at this site. Full access requires a paid subscription, but if you're going to use it frequently, you'll get your money's worth. In addition to the US, it covers trails in Canada, Mexico, and the Caribbean. You'll find backpacking trails, paddling routes, climbing routes, campgrounds, scenic drives, and even surfing breaks.

American Hiking Society: www.americanhiking.org. This site has great information on trails, plus news and other useful information for hikers and backpackers. It's also a good place to check out volunteer opportunities.

American Trails: www.americantrails.org. Great information on all kinds of trails in the US: cycling, horse trekking, and backpacking, mostly through links to other sites.

Trail Peak: www.trailpeak.com. This site has a database of backpacking, climbing, kayaking, and snow sport trails across Canada, and, to a lesser extent, the US and Mexico. The members add trails themselves, so the descriptions vary in length and quality.

Backpacking Lightweight: www.backpacking.net. If you're into the "lighter is better" philosophy, this site is for you. Find out about the latest, lightest gear and how to pack for your adventures. There are also online forums to discuss any issues that come up, or just share your ideas on different trails.

Backpacking Light: www.backpackinglight.com. This print and online magazine provides gear reviews, lightpacking tips, and even a gear shop for lightweight backpacking and camping. Also check out the book *Lightweight Backpacking and Camping* (Beartooth Mountain Press).

Thebackpacker.com: www.thebackpacker.com. This is an online community site featuring trail reviews, gear reviews, articles, and discussion boards. There's also a good section on information for beginners.

Peak to Peak: www.peaktopeak.net. This site provides a wide selection of links to sites across the US and around the world. You can use this as a good starting point to find trails, get in touch with local clubs and organizations, read gear reviews, or find online discussions about wilderness topics.

Appalachian Trail Conservancy: www.appalachiantrail.org. If you're considering a hike on the Appalachian Trail for a day, a week, or six months, this site is a good place to start your planning. It's got the information you'll need on shelters, campsites, shuttle services, and more.

Continental Divide Trail Alliance: www.cdtrail.org. The website has a ton of information about the trail, including which maps you'll need and where all of the access points are. It also contains lots of links for weather reports, emergency frequencies, and other trail necessities.

Pacific Crest Trail Association: www.pcta.org. You'll get some general information about the trail on their website, the most useful of which is probably the trail conditions update. There are also some trip-planning tips and journals from hikers.

International Backpacking Association: www.backpackingfun.com. As the website address suggests, this is mostly a place to find "fun" bits of information, but there's helpful stuff, too. There are articles collected from a variety of newspapers on topics of interest to backpackers. There are also gear lists and cooking tips, and, of course, discussion forums.

Backpacker Magazine: In print or online at www.backpacker.com. This great resource covers trip ideas, trails, gear, technique, and more. There's even stuff just for women, from online forums to gear reviews. If you are regular backpackers and you want to subscribe to just one magazine, this would be the one to get.

Paddling

Paddling.net: www.paddling.net. This is a great resource for all levels of paddlers. It has trip reports, gear reviews, shopping links, articles, and quite an active discussion area. It covers canoeing, sea kayaking, and river kayaking across the US and Canada.

American Canoe Association: www.acanet.org. Despite their name, the ACA also has content for kayakers and rafters. The site has good information about courses you can take through ACA, but their route data is pretty bare bones. There are links to other sites for more detailed information, plus links to clubs and discussion groups.

Paddle Canada: www.paddlingcanada.com. This is the Canadian equivalent of the ACA, offering courses in canoe and kayak paddling at all levels. They also publish a quarterly magazine called *Kanawa* and offer online discussion boards.

Canadian Canoe Routes: www.myccr.com. This site is one of my favorites—good information coupled with a good design make it a pleasure to use. There are articles and trip reports from members, plus a decent collection of recipes to check out. The discussion boards are very active, so this would be the place to discuss paddling trips in Canada with fellow paddlers.

Canoe & Kayak Magazine: In print or online at www.canoekayak.com. This magazine has articles to keep every paddler inspired. Read up on places to go (mostly in the US), techniques, and gear. The online version gives you access to older articles in case you missed out on something that interests you. Their discussion boards are moderately active.

Paddler Magazine: In print or online at www.paddler-magazine.com. This is another good general magazine for paddlers with articles about destinations, trends, and more. The website's "trip finder" is a bit of a misnomer. It actually just provides links to outfitters in different states and countries.

Sea Kayaker Magazine: In print or online at www.seakayakmag.com. This sea kayaker-specific publication provides articles on expeditions and destinations, gear, books, and safety and technique. The website also offers links to various water trails around the US, and links to kayaking clubs and online shopping.

Gear and Clothing

REI: www.rei.com. REI has more than two dozen retail stores across the US, plus an online store for everyone else. They sell gear and clothing from a variety of different suppliers, and have their own house brand as well. The website also offers expert advice on how to choose the right products for your needs, how to care for your purchases, outdoor skills and safety, and packing checklists. As a bonus for couples, they offer a gift registry service so you don't end up getting 15 cappuccino makers on your wedding day when you really wanted a titanium cook set!

MEC: www.mec.ca. Like REI, Canada-based Mountain Equipment Co-op, or MEC, is a co-op retailer where the customers are also owners. MEC has retails stores across Canada and online and catalogue shopping for people in other locations, including the US. They carry gear and clothing for all "self-propelled" activities, including hiking, paddling, rock climbing, and cross-country skiing. They stock a variety of brands, including their own house brand. The website also features an advice section much like REI's, plus links to Canadian outdoor clubs and organizations. They list courses available to improve your wilderness skills, and a "gear swap" website for buying, selling, or trading used equipment.

The North Face: www.thenorthface.com. The North Face makes a wide range of camping products, including tents, backpacks, sleeping bags, clothing, and footwear. You can't buy their products directly from the company, but if you visit their website, you can find a local retailer who carries the product you're looking for.

Mountain Safety Research: www.msrcorp.com. If you've done much camping, chances are you've seen the distinctive MSR logo on fuel bottles everywhere. MSR also makes tents, cookware, hydration gear, and camp towels. You can buy gear directly from their website, or check the retailer listings for a store near you.

GSI Outdoors: www.gsioutdoors.com. If you're looking for outdoor cooking gear and table wear, GSI has it all. They carry a huge range of Lexan products that give your outdoor dining more of a romantic feel. Their selection includes wine glasses, champagne flutes, martini glasses, flasks, a cocktail shaker, and, of course, the Vortex hand-cranked blender.

Design Salt: www.designsalt.com. This company makes the Cocoon system of sleeping gear, designed to layer and zip together for maximum coziness between two people. They also make silk sleepwear so you can get the full lingerie effect even when you're in the woods. You can buy products directly from their website, or check the list of retailers to see if there's one near you.

Lowe Alpine: www.lowealpine.com. As you can tell from the name, Lowe Alpine has its roots in mountain climbing. They make backpacks and clothing for all levels of outdoor enthusiast. They also offer lightweight backpacks specially designed for ultra-light backpackers and adventure racers. You can't buy directly from their website, but you can use it to find a retailer in your area, or an online retailer who carries their products.

Patagonia: www.patagonia.com. Patagonia offers a wide range of clothing for hiking, camping, paddling, climbing, skiing, and traveling, plus a surfer's range as well. Not only are these clothes functional in the outdoors, they're fashionable and even sexy. In addition to clothing, they make a limited selection of backpacks and accessories. You can buy online from their website, or if you prefer to try things on, you can go to one of their retail stores. They also sell their clothing through other retail outlets.

Prana: www.prana.com. Prana's clothing is designed with rock climbing and yoga in mind, so most of it is very form-fitting. Their stuff is designed to be attractive as well as functional, and wouldn't be out of place on the city streets or on the face of a cliff. You can buy online from their website, or use it to find a retailer near you.

Columbia: www.columbia.com. Well-known for its outdoor clothing, Columbia also makes tents, sleeping bags, bicycles, and other gear. Their clothing covers most outdoor activities, and also gets into traveling clothes like skirts and strappy sandals. Their website doesn't offer online shopping, but it will help you to find a retailer that stocks their gear.

Mountain Hardwear: www.mountainhardwear.com. These guys take camping seriously and make quality clothing, tents, sleeping bags, and backpacks. They thrive on innovation, so you may find that they're first on the block to try out new technology or fabrics. Their website will direct you to retailers in your area who carry their products.

Parks

Recreation.gov: www.recreation.gov. This is a good starting point for any US government information on camping and other outdoor activities. This site has recently become the place to make online reservations at National Park campsites. You'll find links to national and state park sites, Forest Service sites, Bureau of Land Management sites, and many others. You can find out about national parks and other recreational passes. There is also access to maps and directions, as well as updated weather reports.

National Park Service: www.nps.gov. If you're planning a trip to a US national park, start here. This site includes driving directions, entrance fees, dates and hours of operation, schedules of events, and park brochures. Unfortunately, you can't actually make reservations from this site. You'll have to go to Recreation.gov (see above) to reserve your campsite.

StateParks.com: www.stateparks.com. Despite the name, this site has information on US national parks, state parks, national forests, recreation areas, national historic sites, and wildlife refuges. The site provides park locations, an overview of the terrain and sights, camping and trail information, and links to other sites for more detailed information.

US Forest Service: www.fs.fed.us. Get information on the national forest of your choice. You'll be able to check weather conditions, fire restrictions, find out the rules for camping and where the campgrounds are, and get all of the latest news. They will also point you in the right direction (via links to other sites) to get your hands on maps of each area.

Parks Canada: www.pc.gc.ca. If you're planning a visit to any of Canada's national parks or marine conservation areas, this is the place to begin. There is a link to their online reservation service where you can book all of your campsites in advance. On the main site, you'll find directions to the parks, fee details, and hours of operation, in addition to general information about the natural features and wildlife in the park.

Cooking

Lipsmackin' Backpackin' by Christine Conners (Falcon 2000). This book garners great reviews for tasty meals and easy-to-follow instructions. It offers lightweight meals that are partially prepared before your trip to save time and fuel. This is a great book for folks with dehydrators. If you're vegetarian, check out the second book in the series, *Lipsmackin' Vegetarian Backpackin'*.

Trail Food: Drying and Cooking Food for Backpacking and Paddling by Alan Kesselheim (Ragged Mountain Press 1998). If you want dehydrated foods to take camping but aren't sure how to start, this book will help you on your way. Once you've mastered the basics, you'll probably want to invest in another cookbook to give you a wider selection of recipes, unless you're a creative cook on your own.

The One-Pan Gourmet: Fresh Food on the Trail by Don Jacobson (Ragged Mountain Press 1993). This book is more focused on eating well on the trail than it is on keeping your load light. However, it does recommend saving weight with unnecessary gear, so the recipes are designed to be cooked in either one pot or one frying pan.

Backpack Gourmet by Linda Yaffe (Stackpole Books 2004). This book also offers recipes for meals you can make in advance or make with dehydrated foods. This one distinguishes itself by having quite fancy dishes to add to your outdoor repertoire. So if you want to make your camping meals a bit more special without wasting time cooking them on the spot, you can use these recipes to do the work in advance. There are vegetarian recipes included, and some veggie options for non-vegetarian meals.

The Leave No Crumbs Camping Cookbook by Rick Greenspan (Storey Publishing 2004). The authors of this book have been teaching cooking to campers for 30 years, so they have a good idea of what the average person can cope with. The result is an easy-to-use cookbook with some innovative recipes. While some require a dehydrator and others will have you packing a camping oven, you'll probably find something in there that's right for your kind of camping.

Freezer Bag Cooking: www.freezerbagcooking.com. A couple of freezer bag enthusiasts have set up this excellent website covering everything you need to know to start packing your camping meals into freezer bags and doing away with cleaning pots and pans and bowls. There is information about equipment, techniques, and, of course, there are recipes. This is about the lightest trail food you can get without relying completely on expensive, freeze-dried meals.

A Fork in the Trail by Laurie Ann March (Wilderness Press 2008). This is another book for the dehydrator enthusiast. Most of the recipes involve cooking and drying at least part of the meal before your trip. Some recipes also use a camping oven. But if you're not put off by the need for gear (and preparation time), you'll find a wide variety of dishes with tempting flavor combinations. Even lunch gets the gourmet treatment here.

Index

About the Author

Writer, camper, and paddler Michelle Waitzman was born and raised in Toronto, Canada, where she worked in TV production for almost 20 years. In 2005, she followed her wander and her *lust* to Wellington, New Zealand, in search of love and the great outdoors (she found both). She now works on the occasional blockbuster New Zealand film project and fine-tunes her lovemaking skills with her partner, Gerhard, on their many "tramping" trips Down Under. Michelle blogs about camping with her partner, and other outdoor misadventures, at loveinatent.blogspot.com. This is her first book.

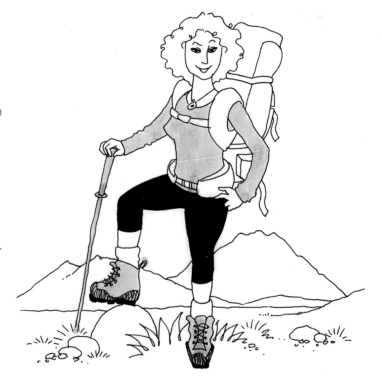

Illustrator Ann Miya lives and works in Santa Cruz, California, where she and her husband share a little compound with Rio the dog and four cats. When not drawing or dog walking, she gardens and practices the ukulele or the accordion. She and her husband recently bought a new tent.